Neurology

PreTest® Self-Assessment and Review

Neurology

PreTest®
Self-Assessment
and Review

Richard Lechtenberg, M.D.

*Director, Central Nervous System Clinical Research
and Development*
Berlex Laboratories, Inc.
Wayne, New Jersey

McGraw-Hill, Inc.
Health Professions Division/PreTest® Series

New York   St. Louis   San Francisco   Auckland
Bogotá   Caracas   Lisbon   London   Madrid
Mexico   Milan   Montreal   New Delhi   Paris
San Juan   Singapore   Sydney   Tokyo   Toronto

Neurology: PreTest® Self-Assessment and Review

1 2 3 4 5 6 7 8 9 0   DOCDOC   9 8 7 6 5 4 3 2 1

ISBN 0-07-051994-3

The editors were Gail Gavert and Bruce MacGregor.
The production supervisor was Clara B. Stanley.
R.R. Donnelley & Sons was printer and binder.
This book was set in Times Roman by Huron Valley Graphics, Inc.

Library of Congress Cataloging-in-Publication Data

Lechtenberg, Richard.
    Neurology : PreTest self-assessment and review / Richard
Lechtenberg.
       p.   cm.
    Includes bibliographical references.
    ISBN 0-07-051994-3
    1. Neurology—Examinations, questions, etc.   I. Title.
    [DNLM: 1. Nervous System Diseases—examination questions.   WL 18
L459n]
    RC343.5.L43   1992
    616.8'076—dc20
    DNLM/DLC
    for Library of Congress   91-29837
                                         CIP

Contents

Introduction

Neurology: PreTest® Self-Assessment and Review is intended to provide medical students, as well as house officers and physicians, with a convenient tool for assessing and improving their knowledge of neurology. The 500 questions in this book are similar in format and complexity to those included in the Comprehensive Part II of the National Board of Medical Examiners examination, the Federal Licensing Examination (FLEX), and the Foreign Medical Graduate Examination in the Medical Sciences (FMGEMS). This book will continue to be a useful study tool for Step 2 of the United States Medical Licensing Examination (USMLE). These questions may also be useful in helping neurology house officers prepare for the certifying examination given by the American Board of Psychiatry and Neurology.

Each question in this book has a corresponding answer, a reference to a text that provides background for the answer, and a short discussion of various items raised by the question and its answer. A listing of references for the entire book follows the last chapter.

To simulate the time constraints imposed by the qualifying examinations for which this book is intended as a practice guide, the student or physician should allot about one minute for each question. After answering all questions in a chapter, as much time as necessary should be spent reviewing the explanations for each question at the end of the chapter. Attention should be given to all explanations, even if the examinee answered the question correctly. Those seeking more information on a subject should refer to the reference materials listed or to other standard texts in neurology.

Neurology

**PreTest®
Self-Assessment
and Review**

The Neurologic Examination and Diagnostic Tests

DIRECTIONS: Each question below contains five suggested responses. Select the **one best** response to each question.

1. Hyperactive tendon reflexes are often an indication of damage to the

(A) spinal cord
(B) peripheral nerve
(C) cerebellum
(D) tendon stretch receptors
(E) muscles

2. Hyporeflexia in the Achilles tendon reflex may be an indication of any of the following EXCEPT

(A) damage to the sensory nerve from the tendon stretch receptor
(B) corticospinal tract damage 1 month prior to the examination
(C) acute transection of the spinal cord at C5
(D) hypothyroidism
(E) diabetes mellitus

3. Rhythmical to-and-fro movements of the eyes may develop with any of the following EXCEPT

(A) looking at a moving striped cloth
(B) riding on a subway train
(C) curare poisoning
(D) phenobarbital overdose
(E) ethanol intoxication

4. Downbeat nystagmus, in which the rapid component of the nystagmus is directed downward and the nystagmus is not gaze-evoked, most commonly develops with damage

(A) in the pons
(B) at the cervicomedullary junction
(C) in the midbrain
(D) in the thalamus
(E) in the hypothalamus

5. Tremor in the hands that is most obvious when the patient is awake but not using the hands usually develops with disease in the

(A) thalamus
(B) substantia nigra
(C) caudate
(D) spinal cord
(E) internal capsule

6. A glove-and-stocking pattern of sensory disturbance with the patient complaining of the sensation of pins and needles over the hands and the feet usually develops with disease in

(A) peripheral nerves
(B) the brachial plexus
(C) the spinal cord
(D) the brainstem
(E) the thalamus

7. Patients complaining of trouble getting out of low seats and getting off toilets often have

(A) poor fine finger movements
(B) poor rapid alternating movements
(C) distal muscle weakness
(D) proximal muscle weakness
(E) gait apraxia

8. A vibrating tuning fork applied to the center of the forehead helps to establish which ear

(A) has a wider range of frequency perception
(B) has a larger external auditory meatus
(C) is lower set
(D) has the longer eustachian tube
(E) has conductive or sensorineural hearing loss

9. Advantages of magnetic resonance (MR) scanning over computed tomographic (CT) scanning include all the following EXCEPT

(A) improved resolution of the cervicomedullary junction
(B) improved recognition of hairline fractures through the temporal bone
(C) improved identification of demyelinating lesions in multiple sclerosis and other demyelinating diseases
(D) improved contrast between gray and white matter structures
(E) elimination of ionizing radiation from the neuroimaging procedure

10. Dysdiadochokinesia is an impairment of

(A) successive finger movements
(B) heel-to-toe walking
(C) rapid alternating movements
(D) tremor suppression
(E) conjugate eye movements

11. Increased sensitivity to sound (hyperacusis) may develop in one ear with damage to the ipsilateral cranial nerve

(A) V
(B) VII
(C) VIII
(D) IX
(E) X

12. Athetosis differs from chorea in being

(A) more symmetric
(B) more forceful
(C) slower
(D) faster
(E) more distal

13. Involuntary twitching at the left corner of the mouth each time a person with left facial weakness tries to blink the left eye suggests

(A) a habit spasm
(B) cerebellar damage producing impaired coordination
(C) aberrant regeneration of the facial nerve
(D) trigeminal neuralgia
(E) focal seizures

14. Spasticity in the right leg usually indicates damage to the

(A) right spinocerebellar tract
(B) left posterior column
(C) right spinothalamic tract
(D) left corticospinal tract
(E) right corticospinal tract

15. The ability to walk along a straight line touching the heel of one foot to the toe of the other is most often impaired with

(A) cerebellar dysfunction
(B) parietal lobe damage
(C) temporal lobe damage
(D) ocular motor disturbances
(E) dysesthesias in the feet

16. The presence of fine twitching movements beneath the surface and wasting of one side of the tongue suggests damage to cranial nerve

(A) V
(B) VII
(C) IX
(D) X
(E) XII

17. Head tilt in a 5-year-old child who seems to be developing clumsiness and gait difficulty suggests

(A) behavior disorder
(B) problems with vision
(C) cerebellar damage
(D) atlantoaxial subluxation
(E) myopathy

18. The patient with an ideomotor apraxia cannot

(A) name his fingers
(B) carry out an imagined act
(C) draw simple diagrams
(D) follow one-step commands
(E) speak fluently

19. With dementia, all the following may be impaired as features of the cognitive disorder EXCEPT

(A) abstraction
(B) memory
(C) coordination
(D) visuospatial perception
(E) orientation

20. Taking a normal, awake person who is lying supine with head slightly elevated (30 degrees) and irrigating one external auditory meatus with warm water will induce

(A) tonic deviation of the eyes toward the ear stimulated
(B) nystagmus in both eyes toward the ear stimulated
(C) tonic deviation of the ipsilateral eye toward the ear stimulated
(D) nystagmus in both eyes away from the ear stimulated
(E) tonic deviation of both eyes away from the ear stimulated

21. Simultaneous irrigation of both external auditory canals with cold water will produce

(A) deviation of the eyes to the right
(B) left beating nystagmus
(C) upward beating nystagmus
(D) upward tonic deviation of the eyes
(E) downward beating nystagmus

22. Rapidly turning the head of a stuporous patient to the right should elicit

(A) horizontal nystagmus in both eyes with the fast component to the right
(B) retraction nystagmus
(C) ocular bobbing
(D) conjugate deviation of the eyes to the right
(E) conjugate deviation of the eyes to the left

23. The Glasgow coma scale measures consciousness by rating parameters that include all the following EXCEPT

(A) orientation
(B) breathing
(C) eye opening
(D) limb posturing
(E) speech

24. The most definitive test for identifying intracranial aneurysms is

(A) MR scanning
(B) CT scanning
(C) single photon emission computed tomography (SPECT)
(D) positron emission tomography (PET)
(E) angiography

25. Myelographic contrast material is usually introduced at the level of the cervical spine if

(A) there is complete obstruction of the subarachnoid space at or below the level of the cervical spine and above the lumbar region
(B) lipid-soluble rather than water-soluble contrast material is to be used
(C) the patient has severe lumbosacral pain
(D) there is substantial risk of transforaminal herniation of the brain
(E) the patient has a type I (adult) Chiari malformation

26. Finding air in the cranial vault after severe head trauma suggests that the patient has

(A) had a severe contusion
(B) had a severe concussion
(C) a skull fracture
(D) had a recent lumbar puncture
(E) a congenital anomaly

27. A useful technique for localizing the site of a cerebrospinal fluid (CSF) leak from the skull uses

(A) CT scanning
(B) radionuclide scanning
(C) MR scanning
(D) pneumoencephalography
(E) electroencephalography (EEG)

28. Large saccular aneurysms are often well visualized on MR scanning of the brain because

(A) thrombus formation in the sac leaves an obvious signal void
(B) high blood flow produces turbulence in the sac
(C) thickening of the aneurysmal wall makes it much denser than cerebral cortex
(D) perisaccular edema enhances contrast
(E) high blood content aggregates iron atoms in a dense locus

29. Positron emission tomography (PET) is useful for

(A) tumor-type identification
(B) establishing the age of an infarction
(C) defining the source of an intracranial hemorrhage
(D) establishing the basis for peripheral nerve damage
(E) examining substrate utilization in the brain

30. The electrocorticogram differs from the electroencephalogram primarily in that it

(A) involves recording directly from the exposed surface of the brain
(B) selectively records abnormal brain-wave activity
(C) uses cup rather than needle electrodes
(D) requires simultaneous cognitive testing of the patient
(E) is used almost exclusively to establish brain death

31. The electronystagmograph (ENG) detects eye movements by monitoring

(A) the heat generated by movements of the globe
(B) action potentials in the ocular motor muscles
(C) the angle between the cornea and the eyelid
(D) changes in orientation of the intrinsic dipole of the eye
(E) EEG activity in the frontal and occipital lobes

32. During relaxation, the normal adult lying with eyes closed in a quiet room will exhibit what type of EEG activity over the occipital and parietal areas bilaterally?

(A) 0 to 3 Hz
(B) 4 to 7 Hz
(C) 8 to 13 Hz
(D) 14 to 25 Hz
(E) 26 to 45 Hz

33. The cerebrospinal fluid (CSF) in healthy adults has all the following characteristics EXCEPT

(A) a total protein content of 60 to 90 mg/dL
(B) gamma globulin constituting 3 to 12 percent of the total protein
(C) 0 to 5 mononuclear cells per cubic millimeter
(D) no red blood cells
(E) a glucose content of >45 mg/dL

34. The most common cause of a positive Romberg sign is

(A) tabes dorsalis
(B) diabetes mellitus
(C) olivopontocerebellar degeneration
(D) multiple sclerosis
(E) vitamin B_{12} deficiency

35. All the following may produce positive Romberg signs EXCEPT

(A) chronic sensory polyneuropathy
(B) syphilitic meningomyelitis
(C) subacute combined systems disease
(D) amyotrophic lateral sclerosis (ALS)
(E) spinal meningioma

36. The magnetic gait of some elderly persons in which posture is slightly flexed, steps are small, turns are accomplished incrementally, and the flow of steps is often interrupted may develop with diffuse damage to the

(A) parietal lobe
(B) temporal lobe
(C) frontal lobe
(D) occipital lobe
(E) corpus callosum

37. Patients with steppage or equine gait have difficulty with

(A) dorsiflexion and eversion of the foot
(B) plantar flexion of the foot
(C) inversion of the foot
(D) flexion at the hip
(E) extension and rotation at the hip

38. With congenital dislocation of the hips, the affected child who has not had corrective surgery will have a gait pattern best described as

(A) shuffling
(B) circumducting
(C) waddling
(D) staggering
(E) steppage or equine

39. The staggering gait typically seen with alcohol intoxication may also develop with intoxication with

(A) amphetamines
(B) cocaine
(C) methylphenidate
(D) barbiturates
(E) aminophylline

40. All the following are characteristic of a cerebellar gait disturbance EXCEPT

(A) wide base
(B) festination
(C) irregular step size
(D) lateral veering
(E) unstable turning

41. Cerebellar gait disorders are likely with all the following EXCEPT

(A) thioridazine (Mellaril) use
(B) chronic alcoholism
(C) olivopontocerebellar atrophy
(D) multiple sclerosis
(E) medulloblastoma

42. Agnosia and dyslexia are similar in that they both occur with defects in

(A) vision
(B) language expression
(C) transcallosal functions
(D) language perception
(E) recognition

43. With damage to the angular gyrus of the dominant parietal lobe, the patient may exhibit all the following EXCEPT

(A) alexia
(B) agraphia
(C) acalculia
(D) finger agnosia
(E) expressive aphasia

44. Narcolepsy is characterized by all the following EXCEPT

(A) hyperphagia
(B) hypnagogic hallucinations
(C) hypnopompic hallucinations
(D) sleep attacks
(E) cataplexy

45. With the sleep fragmentation caused by episodic sleep apnea, susceptible persons are likely to exhibit all the following EXCEPT

(A) morning headache
(B) anorexia
(C) daytime sleepiness
(D) memory dysfunction
(E) personality disturbances

46. Extremely obese persons with hypersomnia and polycythemia typically have arterial blood gases with a chronically

(A) elevated pH
(B) depressed pH
(C) elevated P_{O_2}
(D) elevated P_{CO_2}
(E) depressed P_{CO_2}

47. All the following may produce insomnia EXCEPT

(A) hypothyroidism
(B) depression
(C) sleep apnea
(D) barbiturate withdrawal
(E) stimulant abuse

DIRECTIONS: The group of questions below consists of lettered headings followed by a set of numbered items. For each numbered item select the **one** lettered heading with which it is **most** closely associated. Each lettered heading may be used **once, more than once, or not at all.**

Questions 48–54

For each of the following clinical scenarios, choose the cerebrospinal fluid (CSF) pattern most likely to be found.

	Protein content mg/dL	Glucose content mg/dL	WBC per mm³	RBC per mm³	Opening pressure mmH₂O	Appearance	Gamma globulin % protein
(A)	40	75	3	0	430	clear	8
(B)	300	86	7	0	120	yellow	12
(C)	65	80	8	0	110	clear	17
(D)	95	12	150	3	200	milky	13
(E)	120	65	85	15	300	cloudy	15
(F)	45	78	3	0	130	clear	7
(G)	250	68	20	9808	190	yellow	14

48. A 26-year-old woman with a 7-year history of epilepsy developed a generalized convulsion while shopping. She was taken to an emergency room, but no one accompanying her was aware of the previous history of epilepsy. Because she had a protracted postictal period, numerous investigations were performed over the course of the next hour. Her CT scan was completely normal, but her arterial blood gases revealed a mild acidosis

49. A 72-year-old man was brought to the emergency room (ER) in coma. He had fever and had been observed to have a generalized tonic-clonic seizure just prior to arriving in the ER. His family reported that he had complained of lethargy and cough about 1 week prior to the acute deterioration. On the day of his seizure he had complained of headache and blurred vision. He had had some vomiting early in the day and had become more stuporous as the day progressed. There was no evidence of alcohol or drug use

50. A 19-year-old man noticed discomfort in his ankles within a few days of recovering from an upper respiratory infection. Over the next 7 days he developed progressive weakness in both of his legs and subsequently in his arms. He had no loss of sensation in his limbs, despite the progressive loss of strength. He did not lose bladder or bowel control, but on the tenth day of his weakness he developed problems with breathing and required ventilatory assistance

51. A 40-year-old man was involved in an automobile accident. There was an obvious laceration on his head, and he complained of neck pain. Police at the scene reported that he was unconscious when they arrived, but the patient cannot recall this loss of consciousness. In fact, he cannot remember the accident or events within 10 min prior to the accident. On examination, he had obvious neck stiffness and photophobia. Within a few hours of his arrival at the emergency room he developed vomiting. His lumbar puncture was delayed until after an MR scan could be obtained. The tap was performed 2 days after the accident because the patient still was confused and irritable

52. A 22-year-old woman was brought to the hospital in coma. She had had changes in her behavior characterized by excessive suspiciousness and facetiousness over the month prior to her hospitalization. One week prior to her hospitalization she had visual and auditory hallucinations. Drug testing revealed no apparent illicit drug use. On the day of admission she had a generalized seizure and lapsed into coma. Her MR scan showed unilateral changes in the temporal lobe

53. A 23-year-old woman developed bed wetting that resolved over the course of 2 weeks. One month later she awoke with pain in her left eye. Her vision in that eye deteriorated over the next 2 days. At one point she had little more than light perception in the eye. A neurologic examination revealed that her speech was slightly slurred and rapid alternating movements involving her right hand were poor. She had a positive Babinski sign on the left

54. A 26-year-old woman weighing in excess of 300 pounds complained of headache and blurred vision that began 2 weeks prior to consulting a physician. She had no vomiting or diplopia. Examination of her eyes revealed florid papilledema but without hemorrhages. Her neurologic examination was otherwise entirely normal. She had had a similar problem while pregnant with her fourth child

The Neurologic Examination and Diagnostic Tests

Answers

1. The answer is A. *(Lechtenberg, Synopsis, pp 9–10.)* Deep tendon reflexes are hyperactive with upper motor neuron damage. This means that a motor neuron in the brain or its axon in the spinal cord has been damaged, and the reflex loop in the spinal cord is released from cerebrocortical control. Damage to a peripheral nerve usually produces hyporeflexia, that is hypoactive deep tendon reflex activity. Damage to the cerebellum may produce pendular reflexes, deep tendon reflexes that are not brisk but that involve less damping of the limb movement than is typically seen when a tendon is struck. The patient with a cerebellar injury may have a knee jerk with several swings back and forth of the lower leg when the patellar tendon is struck. The normal knee jerk would have little more than one swing forward and one back. This pendular reflex would be obvious if the leg were hanging down free to move back and forth with the patient sitting on the edge of an examining table. Hyperreflexia of the sort developing with spinal cord disease would be evident regardless of the position of the leg or arm. Repetitive muscle contractions elicited by a single tap on the tendon is called *clonus.*

2. The answer is B. *(Gilman, Essentials, ed 6. pp 55–62.)* Tendon reflexes are affected by a variety of diseases and injuries. With acute transection of the spinal cord, there is an interval of hours or days during which the patient is in spinal shock, and deep tendon reflexes in the limbs are lost. When the reflexes recover from this shock, they will usually be hyperactive, and clonus may be evident in some of them. Damage to the sensory fibers from the tendon stretch organs occurs with any of several diseases, including diabetes mellitus and sarcoidosis. With hypothyroidism, the reflexes may be hypoactive or exhibit other aberrant patterns, but they are generally not hyperactive. The corticospinal tracts carry motor control information from the cerebral cortex to the motor neurons in the spinal cord. Corticospinal tract damage, such as that which would occur with a knife wound to the lateral column of the spinal cord, would produce the same pattern of spinal shock as that exhibited with a more generalized spinal cord injury, but after 1 month there would be no persistent hyporeflexia. The Achilles reflex would be expected to be hyperactive and, indeed, would be expected to be associated with spasticity in the gastrocnemius and soleus muscles of the leg.

3. The answer is C. *(Lechtenberg, Synopsis, pp 5–6.)* Most rhythmical to-and-fro movements of the eyes are called *nystagmus.* These eye movements may have a fast component in one direction and a slow component in the opposite direction. Nystagmus with a fast component to the right is called a *right beating nystagmus.* Many drugs evoke nystagmus, but curare is not one of them. Curare at a high-enough dose will paralyze the eyes, producing ophthalmoplegia. Some drugs, such as phenytoin (Dilantin), may evoke nystagmus at slight overdoses and ophthalmoplegia at massive overdoses in susceptible persons. With phenobarbital and ethanol ingestion, nystagmus may be apparent only when the patient looks to the side or down. This type of nystagmus is called *gaze-evoked.* If the patient has nystagmus on looking directly forward, he or she is said to have nystagmus in the position of primary gaze. Nystagmus elicited by movement in the environment, such as that exhibited by passengers on a train, is a familiar and insignificant phenomenon.

4. The answer is B. *(Lechtenberg, Synopsis, pp 1–12.)* Abnormal patterns of eye movement may help localize disease in the central nervous system. Damage to the pons may produce characteristic conjugate deviations of the eyes. The conjugate eye movements are rhythmical and directed downward, but they lack the rapid component characteristic of nystagmus. This type of abnormal eye movement is called ocular bobbing. A lesion at the cervicomedullary junction, such as a meningioma at the foramen magnum, will produce a downbeat nystagmus with both eyes rhythmically deviating downward with the rapid component of this nystagmus directed downward as well. *Cervicomedullary* refers to the cervical spinal cord and the medulla oblongata. Damage to the midbrain, thalamus, or hypothalamus may disturb eye movements, but downbeat nystagmus would not ordinarily develop with damage to these structures.

5. The answer is B. *(Lechtenberg, Synopsis, pp 1–12.)* The substantia nigra connects with and interacts extensively with the basal ganglia of the brain. The basal ganglia include the caudate, the putamen, and the globus pallidus. The caudate, putamen, and globus pallidus are deep in the brain in the diencephalon, and the substantia nigra is in the brainstem. All of these structures are involved in the regulation of movement. Damage to the substantia nigra, such as that occurring in Parkinson disease, produces the resting tremor described. In the parkinsonian patient, the tremor will abate instantly with the initiation of a directed hand movement. That the patient is awake is an important qualification, because the resting tremor associated with disease of the substantia nigra typically disappears when the patient is asleep. Damage to the thalamus is more likely to produce a sensory disturbance. Damage to the cerebellum may produce a tremor, but damage to that part of the brain more typically produces a tremor that does not worsen at rest but rather becomes more evident with movement of the affected limb. Tremors may develop with spinal cord damage, but they do not follow a typical pattern and do not suggest a spinal cord origin. Damage to the internal capsule may damage connections from motor neurons or from the optic radiation.

6. **The answer is A.** *(Lechtenberg, Synopsis, pp 8–9.)* Sensory disturbances may develop with damage to peripheral nerves, the spinal cord, the brainstem, or the thalamus, but a glove-and-stocking pattern of sensory disturbance is usually seen with lesions that involve peripheral nerves, specifically the nerves extending out into the limbs. The meaning of the pattern is self-evident: sensation is disturbed over the hands and the feet with extension up the arms and the legs being quite variable. The most severe sensory deficit affects the most terminal elements of the limbs. Metabolic or nutritional problems are the usual causes of a glove-and-stocking pattern of sensory disturbance. Diabetes mellitus, thiamine deficiency, and neurotoxin damage, such as that caused by some insecticides, are the commonest causes of these sensory disturbances. Affected persons usually report the sensation of pins and needles in the hands and feet, but with some neuropathies severe pain may develop along with the loss of sensory acuity.

7. **The answer is D.** *(Lechtenberg, Synopsis, pp 7–8.)* With primary muscle diseases, such as polymyositis, weakness usually develops in proximal muscle groups much more than in distal groups. This means that weakness will be most obvious in the hip girdle and shoulder girdle muscles. To get out of a low seat, the affected person may need to pull himself or herself up using both arms. Persons with more generalized weakness or problems with coordination are less likely to report problems with standing from a seated position. Poor rapid alternating movements and poor fine finger movements are both problems usually developing with impaired coordination, such as that which develops with cerebellar damage. With severe weakness in the limbs, patients will do poorly on these tests of function as well. With proximal muscle weakness, the affected person will usually perform relatively well on these tests of distal limb coordination.

8. **The answer is E.** *(Adams, ed 4. p 230.)* The vibrations from a tuning fork placed on top of the head are transmitted through the skull to both ears. Bone

conduction of sound through the skull should be equal in both ears. With sensorineural hearing loss, the patient will hear the midline fork more loudly in the unaffected ear. Sensorineural hearing loss is the deafness that develops with injury to the receptor cells in the cochlea or to the cochlear division of the auditory nerve. With a conductive hearing loss, the vibrations of the tuning fork are perceived as louder in the affected ear. With this type of hearing loss, the injury is in the system of membranes and ossicles designed to focus the sound on the cochlea. With this conductive system impaired, the vibrations of the tuning fork are transmitted to the cochlea directly through the skull. Much like a person with cotton stuffed into the external auditory meati, the patient with the conductive hearing loss has impaired perception of sound coming from around him or her but has an enhanced perception of his or her own voice. This type of tuning fork test is called the *Weber test.*

9.   The answer is B. *(Adams, ed 4. p 17.)* MR scanning does not yet resolve features in dense bone. A small fracture through the petrous pyramid may be obvious on thin (2-mm) cuts through the temporal bone using computed tomography, but the MR scanner will visualize this relatively water-deficient structure poorly. Proton density is critical for MR visualization of brain structures, and water is especially rich in protons. Demyelination, ischemic injury, and inflammation all affect water content, thereby improving contrast on MR visualization of the affected tissues. MR scanning does not use ionizing radiation, but it does use a high-energy magnetic field. The dangers of ionizing radiation are now familiar to physicians and patients alike, but there are few dangers attributed to high-energy magnetic fields.

10.   The answer is C. *(Lechtenberg, Synopsis, p 9.)* Dysdiadochokinesia is usually apparent with cerebellar damage. It is most evident when strength and sensation are intact. Alternately tapping one side of the hand and then the other or tapping the heel alternating with the toe of the foot is the test usually employed to check this aspect of coordination. Multiple sclerosis in adults and cerebellar tumors in children are two of many causes of problems with this part of the neurologic examination. Focal lesions in the nervous system may produce highly asymmetric dysdiadochokinesia. A variety of movement disorders, such as parkinsonism and choreoathetosis, may interfere with rapid alternating movements and give the false impression that the patient has a lesion in systems solely responsible for coordination.

11.   The answer is B. *(Lechtenberg, Synopsis, p 6.)* The facial nerve innervates the stapedius muscle of the middle ear. With paralysis of this muscle, undamped transmission of acoustic signals across the stapedius bone of the middle ear produces hyperacusis. Hyperacusis is an indication that the damage to the facial nerve is close to its origin from the brainstem because the nerve to the stapedius muscle is one of the first branches of the facial nerve. The tensor tympani is controlled by the motor fibers in the fifth cranial nerve. With damage to this nerve the tympanic membrane has some inappropriate slack, but the patient does not usually comment on increased sensitivity to sound in the affected ear.

12. The answer is C. *(Lechtenberg, Synopsis, pp 85–86.)* In addition to involving largely slower movements, athetosis usually has smoother involuntary movements than those typically seen with chorea. Chorea typically involves abrupt, largely discontinuous limb and body jerks. In many cases, the patient exhibits both the more jerking movements of chorea and the smoother movements of athetosis. This combined disorder is called choreoathetosis.

13. The answer is C. *(Adams, ed 4. pp 1081–1084.)* After injury to the facial nerve, regenerating fibers may be misdirected. This is especially common with Bell's palsy (idiopathic facial weakness). Aberrant regeneration is possible only if the nerve cell bodies survive the injury and produce axons that find their way to neuromuscular junctions. Fibers intended for the periorbital muscles end up at the perioral muscles, and signals for eye closure induce mouth retraction. With a habit spasm or idiopathic tic, similar movements may occur, but the movement disorder would not be linked to facial weakness.

14. The answer is E. *(Lechtenberg, Synopsis, p 8.)* Damage to the corticospinal tract or to the cells of origin of these tracts usually produces spasticity, an increased resistance to passive movement across a joint. The corticospinal tracts decussate in the medulla. These fibers synapse with anterior horn cells as they travel down the spinal cord with fibers supplying the legs lying lateral to those supplying the arms.

15. The answer is A. *(Lechtenberg, Synopsis, pp 7–9.)* Walking along a straight line with the heel of one foot touching the toe of the other foot is called heel-to-toe walking, or tandem gait. It is a routine test for ethanol intoxication because alcohol exposure impairs the coordination of gait as governed by the cerebellum. Tandem gait will be abnormal with many other problems, including weakness, poor position sense, vertigo, and leg tremors, but such abnormality in the absence of these other problems suggests a cerebellar basis for the problem.

16. The answer is E. *(Lechtenberg, Synopsis, p 7.)* The hypoglossal nerve innervates the tongue. The fine movements noted under the surface of the tongue with injury to the hypoglossal nerve are called *fasciculations* and are an indication of denervation. They are presumed to occur through hypersensitivity to acetylcholine acting at the denervated neuromuscular junction. Atrophy and fasciculations are likely to occur together and are highly suggestive of denervation of the tongue. This is most often seen with brainstem disease, such as that seen with stroke, bulbar amyotrophic lateral sclerosis (ALS), or with transection of the hypoglossal nerve itself.

17. The answer is C. *(Gilman, Disorders, pp 198–199.)* The combination of head tilt and clumsiness is especially worrisome in young children because this group is at risk for cerebellar tumors, such as astrocytoma or medulloblastoma. Head tilt may be associated with a body tilt and a tendency to fall to the side of the tilt. Children with posterior fossa tumors often complain of early-morning frontal headaches and vomiting.

18. The answer is B. *(Rowland, ed 8. p 4.)* Apraxias are problems with executing activities despite the absence of problems with comprehension, strength, sensation, or coordination that are of sufficient severity to explain the impaired performance. Ideomotor apraxias usually develop with frontal lobe damage. If the patient is asked to act out an activity, such as using an imaginary hammer to drive in an imaginary nail, he will be unable to formulate and perform the actions requested. This type of problem is considered a defect of higher intellectual function and is generally associated with cerebrocortical damage.

19. The answer is C. *(Rowland, ed 8. p 4.)* Dementia is a very broad term for describing cognitive disturbances. To be considered dementia, the intellectual deterioration must be severe enough to interfere with social, occupational, or other routine activities that the affected person had previously performed adequately. Unlike the patient with delirium, the patient with dementia need not have any clouding of consciousness, varying level of awareness, or intermittent agitation. Memory is the function most often first noted to be impaired, but testing of the demented patient may reveal numerous cognitive spheres in which the patient has deficits.

20. The answer is B. *(Adams, ed 4. pp 240–241.)* Caloric stimulation of the ear drives the endolymphatic fluid in the inner ear up or down, depending upon whether warm water or cold water is used. By tilting the head up 30 degrees from the horizontal, the semicircular canal responsible for detecting horizontal head movements is placed in a vertical plane and caloric stimulation drives the endolymph in that canal more effectively than it will the endolymph in the other semicircular canals. The vestibular organ exposed to warm water sends impulses to the brainstem indicating that the head is moving to the side that is being warmed. The eyes deviate to the opposite side to maintain fixation on their targets, but the eye movement actually breaks fixation. A reflex nystagmus toward the ear being stimulated develops as the brain tries to establish refixation and the vestibular signals repeatedly prompt deviation of the eyes contralateral to the warm stimulus.

21. The answer is C. *(Adams, ed 4. pp 240–241.)* Cold water drives the endolymph in the vertically oriented semicircular canals downward. This suggests to the brain or brainstem that the head is tilting upward. Consequently the eyes deviate conjugately downward. Because the head is not actually moving, the eyes are repositioned upward with what is perceived as an upward beating nystagmus.

22. The answer is E. *(Lechtenberg, Synopsis, p 6.)* Conjugate deviation of the eyes to the side opposite the direction in which the head is passively moved is called the oculocephalic reflex. The reflex movement of the eyes keeps them directed toward the same region of space despite movement of the head. The eye movements are essentially a compensation for changes in head position. The patient need not be conscious or even have any useful vision for this reflex to be apparent.

23. The answer is B. *(Lechtenberg, Synopsis, pp 28–29.)* The Glasgow coma scale considers three primary areas of activity: verbal response, motor response, and eye opening. Speech is assessed in terms of whether any is present and whether what is present is comprehensible. The maximum rating of the Glasgow scale is 15; the minimum, 0. This rating scale is most useful for assessing changes in the patient, rather than fully describing the patient's clinical status.

24. The answer is E. *(Toole, ed 4. pp 478–482.)* CT scanning is especially sensitive to intracerebral hemorrhage but not to aneurysms unless they are more than 5 mm across. Even such relatively large aneurysms may not be revealed by CT scanning unless there is bleeding from the aneurysm or distortion of adjacent structures by the aneurysms. Microscopic aneurysms may be localizable on CT only because of the high signal left near the aneurysm by telltale blood. In most cases of aneurysmal bleeding, the angiography is needed to characterize and localize the lesion. The resolution of PET, MR, SPECT, and CT of intracranial aneurysms is too poor to enable surgical correction of the lesion to proceed without demonstration of the aneurysm on angiography.

25. The answer is A. *(Lechtenberg, Synopsis, pp 19–28.)* A cervical or cisternal puncture will help establish the superior extent of a subarachnoid block.

Contrast material introduced during a lumbar puncture will establish the inferior extent. Most myelograms are done with water-soluble contrast material, the principal advantage of which is its uptake from the subarachnoid space and excretion through the kidney. With lipid-soluble contrast agents, the material has to be removed from the subarachnoid space after the myelogram.

26. The answer is C. *(Lechtenberg, Synopsis, p 20.)* Air should not be found in the ventricles or the subarachnoid space even if the patient has had a lumbar puncture. If there has been a skull fracture, it will often be associated with otorrhea or rhinorrhea, the seepage of fluid from the ear or nose. The petrous pyramids and the cribriform plates are especially susceptible to fractures that allow air to enter the subarachnoid space.

27. The answer is B. *(Lechtenberg, Synopsis, pp 20–21.)* A radionuclide introduced into the subarachnoid space by way of a lumbar puncture should be absorbed and excreted without any focal accumulations of material in the head. When a CSF leak occurs, any radionuclide carried along with the leaking CSF will appear as a focal accumulation at the site of discharge. This is usually directly over the cribriform plate or the petrous pyramid, but CSF may dissect along a tear in the dura mater that is relatively remote from the site of an apparent skull fracture.

28. The answer is A. *(Toole, ed 4. pp 478–479.)* MR scanning is not sensitive to blood in vessels unless it is programmed to look specifically at moving elements. How the program analyzes the signal and how the magnetic and radiofrequency waves are manipulated by the imaging equipment is indicated by shorthand notations identifying the type of image obtained from the MR machine. These are designated T1, T2, or otherwise identified by the scanner. The relatively water-depleted clot that fills much of the saccular aneurysm looks like a dark hole on the T2-weighted image. With the resolution available on most currently used machines, the aneurysm must be larger than 6 mm to be obvious.

29. The answer is E. *(Lechtenberg, Synopsis, pp 18–19.)* PET is still a research tool with no clinical advantages over MR or CT scanning. It has special usefulness in determining what materials are used or unavailable for use in specific parts of the brain during various disease states. Seizure activity may be observed in terms of glucose utilization using radioactively labeled glucose.

30. The answer is A. *(Adams, ed 4. pp 26–27.)* The electrocorticogram is nothing more than an EEG performed during neurosurgery without the tissues that usually intervene between the cerebral cortex and the recording electrodes. It is more sensitive than conventional EEG in detecting spike foci responsible for recurrent seizure activity. It is used primarily to direct the neurosurgeon to areas of cerebral cortex that should be resected as part of the management of persistent seizure disorders.

31. The answer is D. *(Lechtenberg, Synopsis, p 23.)* The retina is negatively charged in comparison with the cornea. This creates a dipole that is monitored during ENG studies by electrodes placed on the skin about the eyes. Movement of the most posterior elements of the retina toward an electrode is registered as a negative voltage change at that electrode. The ENG is used primarily to characterize nystagmus and disturbances of eye movements that involve relatively fast eye movements.

32. The answer is C. *(Adams, ed 4. pp 20–21.)* The relaxed adult man or woman exhibits alpha-wave activity at a frequency of 8 to 13 Hz over the posterior aspects of the head. Alpha activity disappears with eye opening and with concentration on mathematical activities. This brain-wave activity should be equally well developed over both sides of the head. As the subject becomes drowsy, the alpha activity becomes less obvious.

33. The answer is A. *(Adams, ed 4. pp 11–14.)* A total cerebrospinal fluid protein (CSF) content in excess of 45 mg/dL in the adult may indicate chronic infection, occult tumor, or other progressive disease even if the affected person is largely asymptomatic. With acute bacterial infection the protein content will usually be elevated, but the glucose content is routinely depressed to less than half the concurrent serum glucose level. After a subarachnoid hemorrhage the CSF protein content increases as the erythrocytes are cleared from the CSF. Extraordinarily high protein levels in the CSF are not unusual with tumors that obstruct the flow of the CSF above the point at which the fluid is collected and with Guillain-Barré syndrome.

34. The answer is B. *(Adams, ed 4. p 95.)* The Romberg sign is a test for position sense in the legs. The patient is asked to stand with his feet together. If he becomes excessively unstable or falls when he closes his eyes, the test is considered positive. This test was originally conceived to screen for patients with tabes dorsalis, the form of neurosyphilis likely to cause posterior column disease. Diabetes mellitus produces a positive Romberg test by disabling position sense at the level of the peripheral nerve.

35. The answer is D. *(Adams, ed 4. p 95.)* ALS is a purely motor syndrome that may produce gait and postural instability but does not interfere with position sense. A spinal meningioma may produce a positive Romberg sign if it overlies the posterior columns and compresses them before it substantially affects other spinal cord elements. Multiple sclerosis (MS) is also a fairly common cause of this sensory disturbance, but cerebellar involvement with MS is so likely that it may be difficult to determine whether the instability is from a defect in position sense or a problem with cerebellar function.

36. The answer is C. *(Adams, ed 4. p 98.)* Gait difficulty in which the patient without basal ganglia disease has flexed posture, small steps, incremental turning, and irregular stepping is often referred to as a *frontal lobe gait apraxia.* An apraxia is a disturbance of action unaccounted for by disturbances in comprehension, strength, sensation, or basic elements of coordination. Obviously, coordination that enables normal gait is disturbed, but this is not a cerebellar disturbance. Similar gait disturbances may occur with basal ganglia degeneration or hydrocephalus.

37. The answer is A. *(Adams, ed 4. p 97.)* With a steppage gait, the foot does not dorsiflex when it is lifted off the ground. The toes remain pointed downward and so the foot must be lifted clear of the ground by exaggerated flexion at the hip. This disturbance results from paralysis of the peroneal and pretibial muscles.

38. The answer is C. *(Adams, ed 4. p 97.)* Because the action of the hip girdle muscles is disturbed with congenital dislocation, the patient compensates by shifting the trunk from side to side. This same pattern develops in some patients with muscular dystrophy and in children with chronic spinal muscular atrophy (Kugelberg-Welander syndrome). With progressive muscular dystrophy, the affected children usually have an associated exaggeration of the lumbar lordosis.

39. The answer is D. *(Adams, ed 4. p 97.)* Alcohol at low doses acts as a mild CNS stimulant, but with intoxication many of the CNS dysfunctions typically seen with barbiturate intoxication become evident. The unstable, reeling, tottering gait typically seen in the drunken person is one such CNS disturbance. Coordination of limb movements is impaired. Truncal stability is disturbed.

40. The answer is B. *(Adams, ed 4. pp 94–95.)* Festinating gait is the short, shuffling gait typically seen with damage to the basal ganglia or substantia nigra, such as that occurring with Parkinson disease. Gait disturbance with cerebellar disease is most often seen with lesions damaging the midline cerebellar structures. The vermis of the cerebellum is presumed to be vitally important in coordination of trunk and limb movements during walking.

41. The answer is A. *(Adams, ed 4. p 95.)* Thioridazine (Mellaril) may produce gait difficulty, but it usually produces a festinating gait, the type of gait characteristic of parkinsonian syndromes. Medulloblastoma is a tumor usually developing during the first few years of life in the vermis of the cerebellum. Chronic alcoholism produces damage in the cerebellum that is most pronounced in the superior anterior vermis. Multiple sclerosis commonly produces demyelination in the cerebellum.

42. The answer is E. *(Adams, ed 4. p 203.)* Both dyslexia (or alexia) and agnosia are problems with recognition. In these disorders, items can be perceived and described and may even be accurately reconstructed, but they cannot be recognized. With dyslexia, the defect is limited to the recognition of printed or written words. *Agnosia* is a much more general term for problems with recognition. These include prosopagnosia, a difficulty with recognizing faces, and simultagnosia, a problem with recognizing a whole item despite the ability to perceive its parts.

43. The answer is E. *(Adams, ed 4. p 386.)* With damage to the angular gyrus of the dominant parietal lobe, the patient may have an aphasia, but this is most likely to be a conduction aphasia or an anomic aphasia, rather than an expressive aphasia. Patients with right-left confusion as well as constructional difficulties, problems identifying which finger is which, and problems with calculations are usually said to have the Gerstmann syndrome. The alexia associated with a lesion of the parietal lobe need not be accompanied by a right homonymous hemianopia.

44. The answer is A. *(Johnson, ed 3. pp 15–16.)* Hyperphagia occurs with some syndromes in which excessive somnolence occurs, but it is not characteristic of narcolepsy. The major characteristics of narcolepsy include sleep attacks, cataplexy, sleep paralysis, and hypnagogic or hypnopompic hallucinations. The cataplexy of narcolepsy is an episodic weakness, often triggered by emotional stimuli. In addition to hallucinations on awakening, the patient may have transient paralysis of limb movements. Hallucinations may occur when the patient is either falling asleep or waking up.

45. The answer is B. *(Johnson, ed 3. pp 17–18.)* Rather than having anorexia, persons with sleep apnea are often obese and have difficulty losing weight. Sleep apnea usually develops with upper airway obstruction during sleep. The patient has intact diaphragmatic and thoracic movements, but upper airway hypotonia produces the obstruction. With airway obstruction, sleep is disturbed.

46. The answer is D. *(Lechtenberg, Synopsis, p 92.)* The combination of obesity, sleep attacks, hypercapnia, and polycythemia is the pickwickian syndrome. Additional problems include right cardiac ventricular hypertrophy and a chronically depressed P_{O_2}. The sleep attacks usually abate when the patient loses weight. The cataplexy and sleep paralysis developing with narcolepsy are not characteristic of the pickwickian syndrome.

47. The answer is A. *(Lechtenberg, Synopsis, p 91.)* If hypothyroidism does produce a sleep disturbance, it is usually hypersomnia, rather than insomnia. Commonly used stimulants that can disturb the normal sleep-wake cycle include ethanol, cocaine, and amphetamines. With barbiturate withdrawal, a normal sleep pattern may not recover for several days after the depressant drug is stopped.

48. The answer is F. *(Lechtenberg, Synopsis, pp 39–48.)* This CSF profile is essentially normal. With idiopathic seizures, the CSF should be normal. Seizure activity does not drive up the CSF protein content or significantly change the cellular content of the fluid. The acidosis observed in this patient is inconsequential, but it is routinely found during the early postictal period after a generalized tonic-clonic seizure.

49. The answer is D. *(Lechtenberg, Synopsis, pp 23–25.)* This man with fever, generalized seizure, lethargy, cough, headache, blurred vision, and progressive stupor probably had an acute bacterial meningitis. Given his age of 72 and history of probable upper respiratory infection, a pneumococcal meningitis is highly probable. The CSF with a bacterial meningitis typically exhibits an elevated protein content, no or few RBCs, an elevated opening pressure, milky or xanthochromic fluid, and a normal or slightly elevated gamma globulin content. If there are relatively few white cells and the CSF protein is not greatly elevated, the fluid may appear clear and colorless. The WBC count will be elevated, and the WBCs in the CSF will consist of both polymorphonuclear cells and lymphocytes. A very low CSF glucose content supports the diagnosis of bacterial meningitis. Tuberculous meningitis, however, produces an atypical pattern of CSF changes, distinct from that caused by other bacterial pathogens and reminiscent of that caused by fungi.

50. The answer is B. *(Lechtenberg, Synopsis, p 100.)* This young man with ascending paralysis with preserved sensation and sphincter control had the Guillain-Barré syndrome. His CSF is largely normal except for its markedly high protein. The CSF is xanthochromic, that is, yellow, because of the high protein content of the fluid. Despite the pattern of weakness suggesting an ascending myelitis, his CSF revealed a normal cell count. That a bacterial meningitis was not responsible for his weakness was supported by a normal CSF glucose content. The CSF protein with Guillain-Barré syndrome may exceed a gram and become so viscous that normal CSF flow patterns may be disturbed.

51. The answer is G. *(Lechtenberg, Synopsis, p 133.)* This man involved in an automobile accident probably had subarachnoid blood associated with his head trauma. This is suggested by his neck stiffness, photophobia, and vomiting. That he had transient loss of consciousness and that there was obvious trauma to his head supports the notion that he suffered enough of a blow to his head to produce intracranial bleeding of some sort. Even if the neuroimaging studies did not reveal any contusion, he could still have a substantial accumulation of blood in the subarachnoid space from damage to vessels in the arachnoid itself. A high CSF protein content and xanthochromia suggest that much of the blood in the CSF has already broken down by the time of the tap. Many RBCs will persist for days with a substantial subarachnoid hemorrhage. The WBC count will be elevated because the subarachnoid blood is irritating and produces a chemical meningitis. The opening pressure may be slightly elevated if there has been much bleeding into the subarachnoid space.

52. The answer is E. *(Lechtenberg, Synopsis, pp 60–61.)* This young woman with progressive behavioral disturbances, hallucinations, seizures, and obtundation probably had a herpes simplex type 1 encephalitis. The CSF with herpes simplex encephalitis often has some RBCs in addition to the primarily mononuclear increase in WBCs. The CSF protein is elevated, but the glucose content is relatively normal with this viral infection. As the CSF protein increases, the percentage that is gamma globulin generally increases. This is not an indication that the problem is an infection, but this increase in total protein and gamma globulin component does occur with infections. The opening pressure may be markedly elevated, but the fluid may remain clear or be only slightly cloudy if the white blood cell count does not increase substantially.

53. The answer is C. *(Lechtenberg, Multiple Sclerosis, pp 70–72.)* This young woman with transient bed wetting (enuresis), optic neuritis, dysarthria, and dysdiadochokinesia probably had multiple sclerosis (MS). Her gamma globulin level exceeded 15 percent of her total CSF protein, as is typical of the gamma globulin component of the CSF in the patient with MS. Further studies on the CSF would probably have revealed oligoclonal banding on immunoelectrophoresis. Her protein content was only slightly higher than normal for her age. That no significant increase in WBCs or RBCs developed argued against her having an encephalomyelitis. The CSF opening pressure and glucose content are normal in most patients with MS.

54. The answer is A. *(Lechtenberg, Synopsis, pp 112–113.)* This woman with headaches, papilledema, and slightly blurred vision probably had pseudotumor cerebri. This idiopathic increase in intracranial pressure usually occurs in obese young women, during pregnancy, or with hypervitaminosis. The extraordinarily high CSF opening pressure associated with pseudotumor cerebri does not produce herniation of the brain, and performing a spinal tap does not place the patient at increased risk for transforaminal herniation. The CSF glucose content, protein content, cell count, and gamma globulin studies in persons with pseudotumor cerebri should all be unremarkable.

Cerebrovascular Disease

DIRECTIONS: Each question below contains five suggested responses. Select the **one best** response to each question.

55. A pure motor stroke is most likely with damage to the

(A) internal capsule
(B) cerebellum
(C) putamen
(D) caudate
(E) amygdala

56. Occlusion of the medial branch of the posterior inferior cerebellar artery (PICA) will damage all the following EXCEPT

(A) corticospinal tracts
(B) nucleus and descending tract of V
(C) nucleus ambiguus
(D) lateral spinothalamic tract
(E) inferior cerebellar peduncle

57. A pure sensory stroke is most likely with damage to the

(A) internal capsule
(B) thalamus
(C) hippocampus
(D) globus pallidus
(E) pons

58. All the following are examples of lacunar stroke syndromes EXCEPT

(A) basilar artery thrombosis
(B) pure motor stroke
(C) pure sensory stroke
(D) clumsy hand–dysarthria syndrome
(E) ataxic hemiplegia syndrome

59. The most common risk factor exhibited by persons with lacunar infarctions is

(A) smoking
(B) hypercholesterolemia
(C) diabetes mellitus
(D) hypothyroidism
(E) chronic hypertension

60. Lacunar infarctions are least likely in the

(A) putamen
(B) thalamus
(C) corpus callosum
(D) corona radiata
(E) cerebellum

61. With the ataxic hemiplegia lacunar syndrome, the ataxia is most pronounced in the

(A) hand
(B) arm
(C) face
(D) tongue
(E) leg

62. Hypertensive encephalopathy may be precipitated in patients taking monoamine oxidase inhibitors with the ingestion of foods containing high levels of

(A) tyramine
(B) tryptophan
(C) serotonin
(D) tyrosine
(E) dopamine

63. Mycotic aneurysms usually develop with

(A) bacterial infections
(B) fungal infections
(C) noninfectious arteritides
(D) endothelial hyperplasia
(E) viral infections

64. With subacute bacterial endocarditis, the most likely cause of focal neurologic deficits is

(A) thrombus formation in the internal carotid artery
(B) vasculitis in the common carotid artery
(C) vasospasm associated with subarachnoid hemorrhage
(D) sagittal sinus thrombosis
(E) vein of Galen malformation

65. Patients with aneurysms producing subarachnoid hemorrhages will have multiple aneurysms in what proportion of cases?

(A) 1 percent
(B) 20 percent
(C) 50 percent
(D) 80 percent
(E) 100 percent

66. All the following are associated with intracranial aneurysms EXCEPT

(A) fibromuscular dysplasia
(B) atrial myxoma
(C) Ehlers-Danlos syndrome (hyperelastosis cutis)
(D) polycystic kidney disease
(E) Hallervorden-Spatz disease

67. The most common type of intracranial aneurysm is

(A) congenital
(B) arteriosclerotic
(C) septic
(D) posttraumatic
(E) paraneoplastic

68. Unruptured aneurysms that produced no symptoms during life are apparent at autopsy in what proportion of the population?

(A) 1 to 5 percent
(B) 10 to 20 percent
(C) 20 to 40 percent
(D) 40 to 80 percent
(E) 100 percent

69. Aneurysms usually become symptomatic

(A) during infancy
(B) during adolescence
(C) between adolescence and 40 years of age
(D) after 40 years of age
(E) with equal probability throughout life

70. Occlusion of the middle cerebral artery may produce any of the following EXCEPT

(A) visual field defects
(B) syncope
(C) hemiparesis
(D) hemisensory defect
(E) aphasia

71. The primitive trigeminal artery may be retained in some adults as a connection between the

(A) internal carotid and basilar arteries
(B) vertebral and basilar arteries
(C) aorta and common carotid artery
(D) ophthalmic and internal carotid arteries
(E) vertebral and lenticulostriate arteries

72. Lacunar strokes account for approximately what percentage of all strokes?

(A) 1 percent
(B) 5 to 10 percent
(C) 15 to 20 percent
(D) 25 to 30 percent
(E) 35 to 40 percent

73. Risk factors for cerebral infarction include all the following EXCEPT

(A) hypothyroidism
(B) hypercholesterolemia
(C) atrial fibrillation
(D) hypertension
(E) smoking

74. Valvular heart disease increases the risk of cerebral infarction especially if the mitral or aortic valves are severely damaged. Efforts to reduce this risk currently include

(A) intracarotid umbrella placement
(B) long-term warfarin
(C) chronic intravenous heparin
(D) repeated courses of tissue plasminogen activator (TPA)
(E) chronic streptokinase

75. In multi-infarct dementia, the extent of intellectual impairment roughly correlates with the

(A) degree of arteriosclerosis in the cerebral vessels
(B) patient's age
(C) number of years dementia has been apparent
(D) number of seizures the patient has experienced
(E) extent of destruction caused by strokes

76. If vertebrobasilar insufficiency is responsible for syncope, the patient is expected to have in association with the syncope some

(A) focal limb weakness
(B) lancinating facial pains
(C) persistent quadriparesis
(D) retrograde amnesia
(E) vertigo

77. Polymyalgia rheumatica is histologically similar to and occasionally appears concurrently with

(A) rheumatoid arthritis
(B) systemic lupus erythematosus
(C) temporal arteritis
(D) psoriatic arthritis
(E) thromboangiitis obliterans

Cerebrovascular Disease
Answers

55. The answer is A. *(Toole, ed 4. p 356.)* Pure motor deficits are especially likely in hypertensive persons with small infarctions called *lacunes*. The pure motor stroke is in fact the most common type of lacunar stroke. The affected person usually has hemiplegia unassociated with sensory or visual deficits. The anterior limb of the internal capsule is the usual site of injury. The lacune is assumed to develop because of an occlusive lesion in a small artery or arteriole supplying the injured structure. It is usually not an isolated problem, and patients with evidence of one stroke during life quite commonly will be found to have multiple lacunes in the brain at autopsy.

56. The answer is A. *(Gilman, Essentials, ed 6. pp 133–134.)* Thrombotic occlusion of the PICA produces the Wallenberg, or lateral medullary, syndrome. In addition to the nucleus and descending tract of V, the nucleus ambiguus, lateral spinothalamic tracts, and inferior cerebellar peduncle, the descending sympathetic fibers, vagus, and glossopharyngeal nerves are often injured with occlusion of this artery. Occlusion of the lateral branch of the PICA produces deficits largely restricted to the cerebellum. The patient with a Wallenberg syndrome has ipsilateral ataxia and an ipsilateral Horner syndrome. The trigeminal tract damage may produce ipsilateral loss of facial pain and temperature perception and ipsilateral impairment of the corneal reflex. The lateral spinothalamic damage produces pain and temperature disturbances contralateral to the injury in the limbs and trunk. Dysphagia and dysphonia often develop with damage to IX and X.

57. The answer is B. *(Toole, ed 4. p 358.)* Pure sensory strokes are most likely in the same persons susceptible to pure motor strokes. With hypertensive injury to the posteroventral nucleus of the thalamus, the affected person will report contralateral numbness and tingling. During recovery from this type of stroke, paradoxical pain may develop in the area of sensory impairment. This paradoxical pain associated with decreased pain sensitivity is referred to as the *thalamic syndrome.* Tricyclic antidepressants are often effective in suppressing much of the discomfort associated with this syndrome.

58. The answer is A. *(Toole, ed 4. pp 356–357.)* Lacunar strokes vary in size from less than 1 mm to 15 mm across. Removal of the infarcted tissue by macrophages produces the characteristic hole, or lacune, from which these strokes get their name. They invariably involve penetrating arteries, but they may arise in either the anterior (carotid) or posterior (vertebrobasilar) systems. There is no therapy that unequivocally affects the probability of developing lacunar strokes. Antihypertensive medications are used if the patient has chronic hypertension, but vascular disease may be too far advanced at the initiation of therapy to affect the likelihood that additional lacunar strokes will occur.

59. The answer is E. *(Toole, ed 4. pp 355–356.)* A risk factor is a statistical connection between a trait and a disease. All the conditions listed are risk factors for some disease, most of them being risk factors for the development of cardiovascular disease. Lacunes occur in patients who have diabetes mellitus or hypercholesterolemia, but they are much more likely to occur with chronic hypertension. With sustained hypertension, lipohyalinosis develops in the walls of the arterioles of perforating vessels in the brain. These arterioles lengthen and develop fibrin deposits, subintimal dissections, and microaneurysms. A lacunar infarction develops if the arteriole becomes blocked with thrombus or if hyperplastic changes in the wall of the arteriole produce occlusion.

60. The answer is C. *(Toole, ed 4. p 356.)* Lacunar infarctions usually occur in several locations in affected persons. Sites notably resistant to the appearance of these injuries include the spinal cord, cerebral cortex, cerebral white matter, and medulla oblongata, as well as the corpus callosum. The putamen, pons, and thalamus are most susceptible to development of lacunar infarctions. These areas are also susceptible to formation of microaneurysms in patients with chronic hypertension.

61. The answer is E. *(Toole, ed 4. p 357.)* Ataxia of the hand, face, and tongue is most likely with the dysarthria–clumsy hand syndrome. With the ataxic hemiplegia syndrome, both the arm and the leg are affected by ataxia and weakness, but the leg is considerably more involved than the arm. The lesion in this syndrome is less well established than in the pure sensory and pure motor syndromes, but it is probably located near the internal capsule or in the ventral pons. The cerebellum is not the site of injury responsible for the ataxia in this syndrome.

62. The answer is A. *(Toole, ed 4. p 359.)* Many cheeses, with the exception of cottage and cream cheeses, have high concentrations of tyramine. The acute elevation of blood pressure induced by tyramine in combination with a monoamine oxidase (MAO) inhibitor may produce intracerebral arteriolar spasm. Cerebral edema, petechial hemorrhages, and ischemic microinfarction develop as the hypertensive crisis persists.

63. The answer is A. *(Toole, ed 4. p 482.)* The name "mycotic" is misleading. It suggests a fungal etiology, but it actually refers to the appearance of the aneurysms, which tend to be multiple. These aneurysms occur with either gram-positive or gram-negative infections, but the responsible organisms usually have relatively low virulence. More virulent organisms producing valvular heart disease are more likely to produce a meningitis or multifocal brain abscess with seeding of infected emboli to the brain.

64. The answer is C. *(Toole, ed 4. p 482.)* Mycotic aneurysms form over the cerebral convexities with subacute bacterial endocarditis. Bleeding from these small aneurysms is largely directed into the subarachnoid space. Cerebral infarction may occur if this subarachnoid blood produces significant vasoconstriction in an artery supplying the cerebrum. The aneurysm appears to develop from an infected embolus originating from the diseased heart valves. Cerebral infarction sometimes occurs because this embolus is sufficiently stable to produce persistent occlusion of the cerebral vessel in which it lodges.

65. The answer is B. *(Toole, ed 4. pp 481–482.)* In the patient with multiple aneurysms, determining which aneurysm is responsible for the intracranial hemorrhage may be quite difficult. In most cases it is the aneurysm that appears largest on angiography that has bled. Persons with multiple aneurysms usually have all accessible aneurysms clipped at the time of surgery. If the site of rupture is inapparent, repeated investigations may be needed to decide on strategy.

66. The answer is E. *(Toole, ed 4. pp 473–474.)* Coarctation of the aorta also occurs with a slightly greater-than-expected frequency in persons with intracranial aneurysms. Atrial myxoma presumably gives rise to aneurysms in the head by injuring intracranial vessels when it sheds emboli. Subacute bacterial endocarditis (SBE) is another entity that induces formation of aneurysms by sending emboli to the head. With SBE, the emboli are presumed to be septic, and the damage they inflict is at least partly due to the bacteria carried in the emboli.

67. The answer is A. *(Toole, ed 4. p 470.)* More than 90 percent of aneurysms are congenital. They are usually berry or saccular aneurysms. Arteriosclerosis is more likely to produce fusiform or giant globular aneurysms. Posttraumatic aneurysms account for fewer than 1 percent of all intracranial aneurysms.

68. The answer is A. *(Toole, ed 4. p 471.)* Aneurysms cannot be viewed as relatively benign because most apparently bleed or cause symptoms by virtue of their size. Of persons dying with subarachnoid hemorrhages, about 90 percent will prove to have one or more aneurysms at autopsy. In about one-tenth to one-fifth of those patients dying with subarachnoid hemorrhages, the aneurysm found will be associated with other aneurysms or an arteriovenous malformation.

69. The answer is D. *(Toole, ed 4. p 471.)* Aneurysms enlarge with age and usually do not bleed until they are several millimeters across. Persons with intracerebral or subarachnoid hemorrhages before the age of 40 are more likely to have their hemorrhages because of arteriovenous malformations rather than aneurysms. Aneurysms occur with equal frequency in men and women below the age of 40, but in the 40s and 50s women are more susceptible to symptomatic aneurysms. This is especially true of aneurysms that develop on the internal carotid on that segment of the artery that lies within the cavernous sinus.

70. The answer is B. *(Toole, ed 4. pp 79–84.)* Syncope associated with middle cerebral artery or internal carotid artery occlusion may occur because of cardiac disease, but should not be ascribed to the cerebral hemisphere damage. If damage is on the dominant side, aphasia of the expressive, receptive, or global type is routine. Hemiparesis and hemisensory deficits are likely to occur together if the occlusion is near the origin of the middle cerebral artery off the internal carotid artery.

71. The answer is A. *(Toole, ed 4. pp 18–19.)* The trigeminal artery is a normal embryonic vessel. It forms as a connection between the internal carotid and the neural arterial plexus that develops into the basilar artery. In the embryo, the trigeminal artery is the principal supply to the hindbrain. Persistence of this vessel in adults usually produces no symptoms.

72. The answer is C. *(Adams, ed 4. pp 643–644.)* Both clinical and autopsy series reveal that about 18 percent of all strokes are lacunar strokes. These are areas of ischemic infarction usually measuring less than a few millimeters across. They develop with relatively small vessel occlusions, but may produce dramatic signs and symptoms if they damage nerve fiber bundles in the internal capsule or the brainstem.

73. The answer is A. *(Adams, ed 4. pp 644–645.)* Although hypothyroidism may adversely affect the lipid profile of susceptible persons, it is not generally regarded as a risk factor for stroke. Atrial fibrillation need not be acute to place someone at increased risk of stroke. Chronic atrial fibrillation is associated with a slight, but real increase in the incidence of cerebral infarction. Hypertension, smoking, and hypercholesterolemia all increase the risk of both myocardial infarction and cerebral infarction, but all three are generally chronic problems extending over years in persons who ultimately have strokes. Cigarette smoking apparently increases the risk of stroke directly by reducing cerebral blood flow and indirectly by reducing the serum content of high-density lipoprotein (HDL) cholesterol, thereby increasing the atherosclerosis developing in vessels supplying the brain.

74. The answer is B. *(Toole, ed 4. pp 39–45.)* The incidence of strokes decreases with oral warfarin taken in sufficient quantity to raise the plasma prothrombin time to about 1½ times the control level. Clots may be blocked with umbrella placement in the inferior vena cava, but this modality is impractical in the carotid. Other anticoagulants have been tried, but chronic administration of intravenous medications is still largely impractical.

75. The answer is E. *(Rowland, ed 8. p 441.)* An estimated one in four patients with dementia has it as a result of vascular disease. For the patient to be symptomatic, the brain must have substantial damage, that damage usually taking the form of infarction secondary to protracted ischemia. The cause of the strokes producing a multi-infarct dementia does not determine the type or severity of dementia that develops. The site of the injury and the amount of brain tissue damaged determine what the patient's signs and symptoms will be.

76. The answer is E. *(Lechtenberg, Synopsis, p 34.)* Signs of brainstem dysfunction usually accompany the loss of consciousness associated with profound vertebrobasilar insufficiency. Signs typically include diplopia, dysarthria, ataxia, dysphagia, tinnitus, or vertigo. This type of vascular problem may develop with severe cervical spondylosis or advanced atherosclerotic disease of the vertebrobasilar system. As a matter of fact, it is relatively rare.

77. The answer is C. *(Adams, ed 4. p 175. Lechtenberg, Synopsis, pp 105–106.)* In both polymyalgia rheumatica and temporal arteritis the patient has perivascular infiltrates with giant cells about cranial arteries, such as the superficial temporal artery. In both syndromes, acute exacerbations may be associated with fever, weight loss, and anemia. Both are usually sensitive to corticosteroid treatment. The pain with temporal arteritis is largely limited to the head, whereas that with polymyalgia rheumatica is widely disseminated.

Epilepsy and Seizures

DIRECTIONS: Each question below contains five suggested responses. Select the **one best** response to each question.

78. Neonatal seizures require emergency investigations that should include

(A) cerebrospinal fluid cultures
(B) minimental status examination
(C) global dementia assessment
(D) token tests
(E) visual evoked responses

79. Most cases of neonatal seizures requiring an antiepileptic medication are treated with

(A) carbamazepine (Tegretol)
(B) ethosuximide (Zarontin)
(C) phenobarbital
(D) divalproex sodium (Depakote)
(E) methsuximide (Celontin)

80. Rapid intravenous infusion of phenytoin is ill-advised because of the risk of

(A) cardiac arrhythmias
(B) respiratory depression
(C) allergic reactions
(D) postural hypotension
(E) amaurosis fugax

81. None of the following is likely to be from seizure activity EXCEPT

(A) bruxism
(B) somnambulism
(C) absence attacks
(D) somniloquy
(E) infantile breath-holding spells

82. Seizures occurring with high fevers are most likely to be transient phenomena with little long-term significance if

(A) they occur in an adult
(B) they occur before 1 year of age
(C) they develop in association with psychomotor retardation
(D) other members of the family have had similar episodes
(E) they occur between 1 and 5 years of age

83. Proconvulsive drugs, which are those that lower the seizure threshold, include

(A) ethanol
(B) aminophylline
(C) barbiturates
(D) streptomycin
(E) digoxin

84. Among children with generalized absence seizures, normal EEG recordings may be exhibited between attacks in as many as

(A) 1 percent
(B) 10 percent
(C) 20 percent
(D) 40 percent
(E) 75 percent

85. The prevalence of epilepsy in the United States is

(A) 0.1 to 0.2 percent
(B) 0.5 to 1.0 percent
(C) 2.0 to 4.0 percent
(D) 5.0 to 7.0 percent
(E) 8.0 to 10 percent

86. Each of the following is likely to cause seizures EXCEPT

(A) subarachnoid hemorrhage
(B) pneumococcal meningitis
(C) cryptococcal meningitis
(D) subfrontal meningioma
(E) multiple sclerosis

87. Generalized absence attacks characteristically exhibit all the following EXCEPT

(A) three per second spike-and-wave complexes
(B) loss of postural tone
(C) staring spells
(D) onset during childhood
(E) sensitivity to ethosuximide therapy

88. The seizure type most commonly occurring in adults is

(A) complex partial
(B) generalized tonic-clonic
(C) generalized absence
(D) simple partial
(E) jacksonian

89. Complex partial seizures may involve all the following segments EXCEPT

(A) an interictal period
(B) an aura
(C) an ictus
(D) a postictal period
(E) a jacksonian march

90. With tonic-clonic status epilepticus, the patient is at risk of dying from all the following EXCEPT

(A) hyperthermia
(B) dehydration
(C) transforaminal herniation
(D) cardiac arrhythmias
(E) renal failure

91. Most physicians recommend using a high dose of intravenous benzodiazepine as part of the management of status epilepticus because of its

(A) ability to suppress seizure activity for more than 24 h after one injection
(B) lack of respiratory depressant action
(C) rapid onset of action after intravenous administration
(D) lack of hypotensive effects
(E) lack of dependence on hepatic function for its metabolism and clearance

DIRECTIONS: The group of questions below consists of lettered headings followed by a set of numbered items. For each numbered item select the **one** lettered heading with which it is **most** closely associated. Each lettered heading may be used **once, more than once, or not at all.**

Questions 92–96

For each of the following clinical scenarios, choose the seizure type from the list below that best explains the patient's complaints.

(A) Generalized tonic-clonic
(B) Generalized absence
(C) Complex partial
(D) Simple partial motor
(E) Simple partial sensory
(F) Jacksonian march
(G) Psychomotor status
(H) Tonic-clonic status
(I) Pseudoseizures
(J) Myoclonic

92. A 37-year-old man developed involuntary twitching movements in his left thumb. Within 30 s he noticed that the twitching had spread to his entire left hand and involuntary movements had developed in his left forearm and the left side of his face. He could not recall what happened subsequently, but his wife reported that he fell down, and the entire left side of his body appeared to be twitching. He appeared to be unresponsive for about 3 min and confused for another 15 min. During the episode he bit his tongue and wet his pants

93. A 17-year-old boy reported involuntary jerking movements in his arms when he awakened. This occurred during the day after a nap, as well as in the morning after a full night's sleep. Over the next few months he developed similar jerks during the day even when he had been awake for several hours. He did not lose consciousness with these muscle jerks, but did occasionally fall. On one occasion, jerks in his legs resulted in a fall during which he fractured his wrist

94. A 21-year-old man reported several episodes over the previous 4 years during which he lost consciousness. He had no warning of the impending episode, and with each episode he injured himself. Observers told him that he abruptly developed a blank stare and stopped talking. His body became stiff and he arched his back. After several seconds of this type of posturing, he started shaking his arms and legs violently. During one of these episodes, he dislocated his right shoulder. He routinely bit his tongue and urinated in his pants

95. A 25-year-old woman was fired from her job after she misplaced papers vital for the company. She had had recurrent episodes for several years during which she did nonsensical activities, such as burying her plates in the back-

yard, hiding her underwear, and discarding her checkbook. She did not recall what she had done after performing these peculiar activities. She had been referred for psychotherapy, but the episodes had only become more frequent after she had been started on thioridazine (Mellaril). Her husband observed one episode and noted that she was unresponsive for about 5 min and confused for at least an hour. She did not fall down or remain immobile during the episodes. As the episodes became more frequent, she noticed that she would develop an unpleasant taste in her mouth, reminiscent of motor oil, just before an episode

96. A 7-year-old boy was inattentive in class repeatedly during the day and was failing all of his subjects. His teacher noticed that he would have frequent staring spells and would occasionally smack his lips. He never fell or wet his pants, but during the brief spells he would not respond when his name was called. His mother had observed similar episodes for 3 years but had simply thought that the child was daydreaming

Epilepsy and Seizures
Answers

78. The answer is A. *(Johnson, ed 3. p 24.)* Visual evoked responses can be recorded from the newborn, but they are not useful as part of the emergency evaluation of the infant with neonatal seizures. CSF cultures are important with neonatal seizures because a bacterial or fungal meningitis may be rapidly fatal unless promptly treated. Additional tests appropriate with neonatal seizures include serum electrolytes, ammonia, and glucose and arterial blood gases. Urine screens should be performed to check for amino or other organic acids. CT or MR scanning of the infant's head is appropriate if the neonate is adequately stable.

79. The answer is C. *(Johnson, ed 3. p 25.)* Despite the many problems associated with phenobarbital use in children, it is still the drug of choice for most neonatal seizure disorders simply because a safer but equally effective medication is unavailable. Initially the infant is routinely given 20 mg/kg with a maintenance dose usually of 3 to 4 mg/kg per day being given subsequently in divided doses as two or three injections daily. Respiratory depression and hypotension must be watched for as complications of this drug in the neonate. Developmental delays may also occur in the infant treated with phenobarbital, but leaving the infant untreated is not a safe alternative. Status epilepticus may develop if the child is on no medication, and that is a potentially lethal problem.

80. The answer is A. *(Lechtenberg, Seizure, p 177.)* Intravenous administration of phenytoin can be accomplished without producing cardiac arrhythmias, but this usually requires an infusion rate of less than 50 mg/min in the adult and of less than 3 mg/kg/min in infants and children. Intravenous loading with phenytoin is appropriate when the patient is actively in seizure and seizures themselves have become a life-threatening problem. Most physicians monitor the ECG while infusing the phenytoin. This is standard practice, but it does little to avert complications. The physician will be aware of a cardiac complication sooner with monitoring than without, but managing the cardiac problem is a difficult problem regardless of how quickly it is detected. Fortunately, this is an uncommon complication of phenytoin infusion. Patients given intravenous phenytoin must be closely watched for hypotension and respiratory depression.

81. The answer is C. *(Lechtenberg, Synopsis, p 48.)* Almost any motor activity may represent a seizure phenomenon, but absence attacks are by definition from generalized or partial seizure activity. Phenomena such as somnambulism (sleep walking), somniloquy (sleep talking), night terrors, and bruxism (tooth grinding) arouse concern that a seizure may be responsible for the observed activity because sleep is especially likely to provoke seizures. Esophageal reflux, breath-holding spells, and shuddering are often seen during infancy and also arouse concerns that seizures are occurring, but they are not epileptic phenomena. Generalized absence attacks are usually associated with three per second spike-and-wave discharges on the EEG of the patient during the seizures.

82. The answer is E. *(Lechtenberg, Synopsis, p 43.)* Febrile seizures are considered simple or complex. Simple seizures are associated with less long-term morbidity than the complex seizures. A febrile seizure is simple if it occurs between 1 and 5 years of age, if it is a generalized seizure, if it lasts less than 15 min, if it occurs in the absence of other neurologic signs, and if the child experiencing the seizure is the only member of the family to have seizures. If an adult has seizures associated with a high fever, he or she must be assumed to have meningitis or encephalitis until proved otherwise. The adult brain is not as vulnerable to systemic temperature elevations as is the infant brain.

83. The answer is B. *(Lechtenberg, Synopsis, p 45.)* Ethanol and barbiturates lower the seizure threshold as their levels in the brain fall. Consequently they may produce withdrawal seizures as part of what is usually referred to as a *rebound effect.* Aminophylline, cocaine, amphetamines, and methaqualone all lower the seizure threshold as they accumulate in the brain.

84. The answer is C. *(Adams, ed 4. p 2.)* A normal EEG recording does not indicate that episodes of altered consciousness are from nonepileptic problems. Children with generalized seizure disorders may have completely normal EEGs between attacks but entirely characteristic recordings during the episodes of altered consciousness. This is even more so for adults with generalized seizure disorders, with as many as 40 percent of patients with generalized tonic-clonic seizures exhibiting normal EEGs between authentic seizure episodes. Detection of a seizure disorder in those with normal interictal records is greatly simplified by continuous EEG monitoring. A 24-h ambulatory recording may reveal very circumscribed spike-and-slow-wave discharges associated with episodes of altered consciousness.

85. The answer is B. *(Lechtenberg, Seizure, p 3.)* The prevalence of epilepsy is higher in Europe and Japan than it appears to be in the United States, but this may be because of better reporting rather than more disease. Epilepsy is defined as a tendency to have recurrent seizures. Isolated seizures occur in more than 1 in 200 persons in the United States, but these individuals do not necessarily have epilepsy.

86. The answer is E. *(Lechtenberg, Multiple Sclerosis, p 73.)* Demyelinating diseases usually do not produce seizures. Seizures are a disorder of gray matter, and so diseases strictly of white matter would not be expected to cause seizures. While there are several demyelinating diseases (e.g., progressive multifocal leukoencephalopathy and metachromatic leukodystrophy) that routinely do produce seizures, multiple sclerosis should never be considered the probable cause of seizure activity.

87. The answer is B. *(Johnson, ed 3. pp 33–34.)* During a generalized absence seizure, the affected child may exhibit slight movement of the eyes or the mouth. Otherwise there is little evidence of seizure activity. Because the children do not lose postural tone, they do not fall during the attacks. Seizures may occur several times a month or several times a day.

88. The answer is A. *(Lechtenberg, Seizure, pp 41–42.)* Partial seizures with complex symptomatology are the most common type of partial seizures, but generalized seizures occur more commonly than partial seizures in children. Adults developing partial seizures of any type between the ages of 30 and 60 have a high probability of having a brain tumor as the basis for the seizure activity. Many complex seizures arising with or without a structural lesion as their basis originate in the temporal lobe.

89. The answer is E. *(Lechtenberg, Seizure, pp 42–43.)* Many patients with complex partial seizures have a preseizure phenomenon, the aura, that alerts them to an impending seizure. The ictus is that part of the seizure during which the characteristic features of the seizure are most evident. During the postictal period, the patient has more nonspecific confusion, agitation, and exhaustion. Between distinct seizure episodes—that is during the interictal period—the patient may exhibit personality traits or behavior patterns that are much more common in persons with a specific seizure type than in those who are not epileptic.

90. The answer is C. *(Lechtenberg, Synopsis, p 48.)* If the patient has an expanding intracranial lesion that is causing the status epilepticus, transforaminal herniation may be present, but status epilepticus per se does not cause brain damage that will produce edema and lead to herniation. Extensive muscle damage does occur with status, and this produces myoglobinuria. The renal tubule becomes obstructed with a massive load of myoglobin, and renal failure may develop. Autonomic problems are fairly common causes of death in patients with status epilepticus.

91. The answer is C. *(Lechtenberg, Synopsis, pp 49–50.)* Until recently the most popular benzodiazepine for use in status epilepticus was diazepam

(Valium). It had a rapid onset of action, but it was cleared relatively quickly. Patients needed additional medications, such as phenytoin, to protect them from recurrent seizure activity as early as 20 min after the diazepam injection. A longer-acting benzodiazepine, lorazepam (Ativan), is gaining in popularity because it is rapid-acting like diazepam but more slowly cleared from the body.

92–96. The answers are: 92-F, 93-J, 94-A, 95-C, 96-B. *(Lechtenberg, Seizure, pp 36–46.)* With a Jacksonian march, or sequential seizure, the patient develops focal seizure activity that is primarily motor and spreads. This type of seizure often secondarily generalizes, at which point the patient loses consciousness and may have a generalized tonic-clonic seizure. The hand is a common site for the start of a Jacksonian march. The face may be involved early because the thumb and the mouth are situated near each other on the motor strip of the cerebral cortex.

Myoclonic seizures may be generalized or partial seizures. They are most commonly seen in the epilepsy syndrome of young people called *benign juvenile myoclonic epilepsy (BJME)*. Unlike sleep myoclonus, the episodes occur when the affected person wakes up, rather than when he or she is falling asleep. Myoclonic jerks may be triggered by light flashes or loud sounds. BJME accounts for 4 percent of all cases of epilepsy. More than half of those with BJME have generalized tonic-clonic seizures, as well as myoclonic seizures.

With generalized tonic-clonic seizures, the EEG develops abnormalities all over the cortex simultaneously. The patient may recall a strange sensation before the attack, but it is equally likely that no premonitory sign or aura will occur. Partial seizures may secondarily generalize to this type of seizure. If the patient has frequent generalized tonic-clonic seizures, he or she will be at high risk for a variety of injuries, such as dislocated shoulders, broken bones, and head trauma. Patients with this type of seizure always lose consciousness during the attack and may be confused for minutes or hours after the ictus, the most obvious segment of the seizure.

Complex partial seizures may be mistaken for a psychiatric problem, especially if the partial seizures do not generalize and produce a tonic-clonic seizure. This patient had a typical aura involving an unpleasant smell or taste. These were once called "uncinate fits," because they were ascribed to abnormal activity in the uncus of the temporal lobe. Complex partial seizures may arise from a focus of abnormal electrical activity in the temporal lobe but do not invariably arise from a temporal lobe focus.

Generalized absence attacks have no aura and no postictal period. The affected child has no warning that an attack is about to occur and is usually unaware that one has occurred unless it is more than a few seconds long. In fact, generalized absence seizures are most often only a few seconds long.

Headache and Facial Pain

DIRECTIONS: Each question below contains five suggested responses. Select the **one best** response to each question.

97. Pain localized about one eye develops for several weeks or months each year and occurs most prominently at night within a few hours of falling asleep. This is highly suggestive of

(A) classic migraine
(B) cluster headache
(C) common migraine
(D) trigeminal neuralgia
(E) sinusitis

98. Pain originating from stimuli about the forehead, orbit, anterior fossa, middle fossa, and the upper surface of the tentorium cerebelli is mediated by signals along

(A) the ophthalmic division of the trigeminal nerve
(B) the maxillary division of the trigeminal nerve
(C) the mandibular division of the trigeminal nerve
(D) the sensory division of C1
(E) sensory divisions of the ninth and tenth cranial nerves

99. All the following are characteristic of migraine headache EXCEPT

(A) familial occurrence
(B) unilateral pattern
(C) throbbing pain
(D) periodic pattern
(E) worsening with age

100. Which of the following is more apparent in classic than in common migraine?

(A) Photophobia
(B) Response to oral ergotamine
(C) A familial pattern
(D) Hemicranial pain
(E) Nausea

101. The visual defect associated with classic migraine is usually

(A) homonymous
(B) centrocecal
(C) sickle-shaped
(D) binasal
(E) bitemporal

102. The pattern of the scotoma associated with classic migraine suggests that it originates from a disturbance of the

(A) retina
(B) optic nerves
(C) optic chiasm
(D) optic radiation
(E) occipital cortex

103. Vertebrobasilar migraine differs from classic migraine in the

(A) sex of the persons most often affected
(B) resistance of the visual system to involvement
(C) severity of symptoms
(D) duration of the aura
(E) sequence of neurologic deficits and headache

104. The nerve most often symptomatic with ophthalmoplegic migraine is cranial nerve

(A) III
(B) IV
(C) VI
(D) VII
(E) IX

105. In families with hereditary hemiplegic migraine, the pattern of inheritance for the disturbance is usually

(A) autosomal recessive
(B) autosomal dominant
(C) sex-linked recessive
(D) maternally linked (mitochondrial)
(E) highly variable

106. All the following are typically found with temporal arteritis EXCEPT

(A) elevated erythrocyte sedimentation rates
(B) involvement of both men and women
(C) pain localized to one or both temporal areas
(D) improvement with advancing age
(E) headaches that persist for weeks or months

107. A 43-year-old woman complains of lancinating pains radiating into the right side of her jaw. This discomfort has been present for more than 3 years and has started occurring more than once a week. The pain is paroxysmal and routinely triggered by cold stimuli, such as ice cream and cold drinks. She has sought relief with multiple dental procedures and has already had two teeth extracted. Multiple neuroimaging studies reveal no structural lesions in her head. Assuming there are no contraindications to the treatment, a reasonable next step would be to prescribe

(A) clonazepam (Klonopin) 1 mg orally (PO) three times daily
(B) diazepam (Valium) 5 mg PO two times daily
(C) divalproex sodium (Depakote) 250 mg PO three times daily
(D) indomethacin (Indocin) 10 mg PO three times daily
(E) carbamazepine (Tegretol) 100 mg PO three times daily

108. The distinct episodes of pain associated with trigeminal neuralgia usually persist

(A) seconds
(B) minutes
(C) hours
(D) days
(E) weeks

109. Symptomatic trigeminal neuralgia may arise with any of the following problems EXCEPT

(A) multiple sclerosis
(B) Tolosa-Hunt syndrome
(C) basilar artery aneurysm
(D) acoustic schwannoma
(E) posterior fossa meningioma

110. The division of the trigeminal nerve most likely to be symptomatic with tic douloureux is the

(A) ophthalmic division
(B) maxillary division
(C) mandibular division
(D) medial component of the ophthalmic
(E) lateral component of the ophthalmic

111. Both trigeminal neuralgia and atypical facial pain involve pain that may be

(A) lancinating
(B) paroxysmal
(C) associated with anesthetic patches
(D) abolished with resection of the gasserian ganglion
(E) unilateral

Headache and Facial Pain

Answers

97. The answer is B. *(Adams, ed 4. p 135.)* The pain of cluster headache is usually described as originating in the eye and spreading over the temporal area as the headache evolves. Men are more often affected, and extreme irritability may accompany the headache. The pain usually abates in less than an hour. Affected persons routinely have autonomic phenomena associated with the headache that include unilateral nasal congestion, tearing from one eye, conjunctival injection, and pupillary constriction. The autonomic phenomena are on the same side of the face as the pain.

98. The answer is A. *(Adams, ed 4. p 136.)* The first division of the trigeminal nerve has so widespread a distribution that the site where pain is perceived may be misleading. Irritation of the tentorium cerebelli from a meningioma may be perceived as pain over the eyes. Much of the posterior fossa is in fact supplied by cervical sensory roots. The tentorium cerebelli roughly demarcates the intracranial regions supplied by the trigeminal from those supplied by cervical nerves.

99. The answer is E. *(Adams, ed 4. p 138.)* Migraine headaches do occur in the elderly, but there is some decrease in the frequency and severity of attacks in most persons as they get older. Fatigue, irritability, and easy distractibility often develop before a migraine attack at any age. Affected persons usually also have hypersensitivity to light and noise during the attack. The pain is usually limited to one side of the head and is throbbing in character. Nausea and vomiting develop with the pain in some types of migraine.

100. The answer is C. *(Adams, ed 4. p 138.)* Familial patterns are not unusual with either classic or common migraine, but with classic migraine, that is migraine with aura, the probability that another family member will have a similar problem approaches 80 percent. Nausea is likely with both classic and common migraine, but vomiting is much more routine with classic migraine. The common migraine is more often unheralded by premonitory signs, such as a scintillating scotoma, than is the classic migraine.

101. The answer is A. *(Adams, ed 4. p 138.)* The blind spot, or scotoma, that may develop as part of the aura of a classic migraine attack will involve the same visual field in both eyes. This defect usually changes over the course of minutes. It typically enlarges and may intrude upon central vision. The margin of the blind spot is often scintillating or dazzling. If this margin has a pattern like the battlement of a castle, it is called a *fortification spectrum*, or *teichopsia*.

102. The answer is E. *(Adams, ed 4. p 138.)* Homonymous hemianopic defects of the sort developing during the aura of a classic migraine indicate an irritative lesion affecting one part of the occipital cortex in one hemisphere of the brain. The changes in the scotoma over the course of minutes indicates that the irritative phenomenon sets off a cascade of events in the visual cortex that temporarily disturbs vision in a progressively larger area. Other focal neurologic phenomena may precede classic migraine, the most common being tingling of the face or hand, mild confusion, transient hemiparesis, and ataxia.

103. The answer is C. *(Adams, ed 4. p 139.)* As with classic migraine, with vertebrobasilar migraine women are more susceptible than men, disturbances of vision are common, the aura usually resolves within 10 to 30 min, and the headache invariably follows, rather than precedes, the neurologic deficits; however, the character and severity of neurologic deficits associated with vertebrobasilar migraine are distinct. The visual change may evolve to complete blindness. Irritability may develop into frank psychosis. Rather than a mild hemiparesis, the patient may have a transient quadriplegia. Stupor, syncope, and even coma may appear and persist as problems for hours.

104. The answer is A. *(Adams, ed 4. p 139.)* With ophthalmoplegic migraine, the patient usually exhibits transient ptosis and oculomotor paresis with normal pupillary function. The oculomotor dysfunction may persist during the headache and be evident for hours or days after the headache remits. Ptosis may in fact be irreversible after an attack.

105. The answer is B. *(Adams, ed 4. p 139.)* Hemiplegic migraine is associated with an increased incidence of persistent neurologic deficits in young women. Either sex may be affected and attacks occur at all ages. Its relationship to common and classic migraine is unestablished.

106. The answer is D. *(Adams, ed 4. p 141.)* Temporal arteritis is largely nonexistent in persons under 50 years of age and rare in those under 60. Loss of vision in one eye may occur with this inflammatory disorder. More generalized pain and fatigue is not at all uncommon, and many patients exhibit persistent fevers and progressive weight loss. Corticosteroids are the treatment of choice.

107. The answer is E. *(Lechtenberg, Synopsis, pp 114–115.)* This woman probably has trigeminal neuralgia (tic douloureux). The treatment options for this facial pain disorder include carbamazepine (Tegretol). Neutropenia routinely occurs with chronic carbamazepine use, thereby making it inadvisable in a patient with an already low WBC count. Although carbamazepine is a potent antiepileptic medication, other antiepileptic medications, such as phenobarbital and divalproex sodium (Depakote), are usually ineffective in blunting the pain. Phenytoin (Dilantin) is another antiepileptic useful in the management of trigeminal neuralgia. Analgesics and anti-inflammatory drugs, such as indomethacin (Indocin), are notably ineffective in managing this disorder.

108. The answer is A. *(Adams, ed 4. p 150.)* The lancinating pains of tic douloureux may occur many times an hour, but each paroxysm lasts only a second or two. The pain may be triggered by eating or drinking, in which case the patient may rapidly lose weight before the pain is brought under control. Trigger zones for the pain may be limited to inside the mouth or to relatively small patches of skin on the face. Despite the severity of the pain and the localizability of the trigger zones, sensory deficits on the face or in the mouth are notably absent in this syndrome.

109. The answer is B. *(Adams, ed 4. pp 150–151.)* The Tolosa-Hunt syndrome is a presumably inflammatory disorder that produces opthalmoplegia associated with headache and loss of sensation over the forehead. Pupillary function is usually spared, and the site of pathology is believed to be in the superior orbital fissure or the cavernous sinus. Multiple sclerosis, basilar artery aneurysms, acoustic schwannomas, and posterior fossa meningiomas may cause trigeminal dysfunction by direct impingement on the nerve or by demyelination of the sensory pathway in the brainstem.

110. The answer is C. *(Adams, ed 4. pp 150–151.)* The mandibular and maxillary divisions may be simultaneously affected in trigeminal neuralgia, but the mandibular is much more commonly affected alone. The ophthalmic division is the component least likely to be involved. Regardless of which division is most symptomatic, the pain is usually unilateral and highly focal.

111. The answer is E. *(Adams, ed 4. pp 150–151.)* Although atypical facial pain is often bilateral, it may be unilateral and fairly limited in its distribution. The cheek, nose, or zygomatic regions are often affected by this idiopathic pain syndrome. The pain is often sensitive to antidepressant medication, a characteristic that has led some to suggest that the syndrome is invariably caused by depression.

Traumatic and Occupational Injuries

DIRECTIONS: Each question below contains five suggested responses. Select the **one best** response to each question.

112. Keyboard operators and typists are especially susceptible to injury of the

(A) axillary nerve
(B) median nerve
(C) ulnar nerve
(D) radial nerve
(E) long thoracic nerve

113. A gunshot wound to the upper arm causing shock-wave damage to the median nerve may leave the patient with

(A) easily provoked pain in the hand
(B) weakness on wrist extension
(C) atrophy in the first dorsal interosseous muscle
(D) numbness over the fifth digit
(E) radial deviation of the hand

114. Blunt trauma to the elbow may lead to the development of

(A) wristdrop
(B) weakness of the abductor pollicis brevis
(C) clawhand or benediction sign
(D) ulnar deviation of the hand
(E) poor pronation of the forearm

115. When a person works in an environment in which loud noises are routine, such as an aircraft testing facility, ear defenders must be worn to protect against loss of hearing and the development of

(A) vertigo
(B) tinnitus
(C) ataxia
(D) diplopia
(E) oscillopsia

116. A young man fractured his humerus in an automobile accident. As the pain from the injury subsided he noticed that he had weakness on attempted flexion at the elbow. He developed paresthesias over the radial and volar aspects of the forearm. During the accident he probably injured his

(A) suprascapular nerve
(B) long thoracic nerve
(C) musculocutaneous nerve
(D) radial nerve
(E) median nerve

117. A 37-year-old alcoholic man awoke with clumsiness of his right hand. Neurologic examination revealed poor dorsiflexion of the hand at the wrist. He most likely injured his

(A) median nerve
(B) brachioradialis nerve
(C) musculocutaneous nerve
(D) radial nerve
(E) ulnar nerve

118. Computed tomography (CT) of the brain may fail to reveal a small subdural hematoma if

(A) the lesion is subacute and the subdural collection is isodense with the brain
(B) the hematoma extends into the brain from the subdural space
(C) the resolution of the CT machine is greater than 2 mm
(D) the subdural hematoma is less than 4 h old
(E) the patient has extensive cerebral atrophy

Questions 119–122

A 16-year-old boy was struck on the side of the head by a bottle thrown by a friend involved in a prank. He appeared dazed for about 30 s but was apparently lucid for several minutes before he abruptly became stuporous. Limbs on the side of his body opposite the site of the blow were more flaccid than those on the same side as the injury. On arrival in the emergency room 25 min after the accident, he was unresponsive to painful stimuli. His pulse was 40 beats per minute with an ECG revealing no arrhythmias. His blood pressure in both arms was 170/110 mmHg. Although papilledema was not evident in his fundi, he had venous distention and absent pulsations of the retinal vasculature.

Answer the following questions with this clinical scenario in mind.

119. The best explanation for this young man's evolving clinical signs is

(A) a seizure disorder
(B) a cardiac conduction defect
(C) increased intracranial pressure
(D) sick sinus syndrome
(E) communicating hydrocephalus

120. The wisest management over the next 4 h for this young man who has been struck on the head is

(A) craniotomy
(B) antihypertensive medication
(C) transvenous pacemaker placement
(D) ventriculoperitoneal shunt
(E) antiepileptic medication

121. MR scanning of this young man's head within the first few hours of injury should reveal

(A) a normal brain
(B) intracerebral hematoma
(C) temporal lobe contusion
(D) subarachnoid hemorrhage
(E) epidural hematoma

122. CT scanning of this young man's head within 2 h of the injury should reveal

(A) a normal brain
(B) a lens-shaped density over the frontal lobe
(C) increased CSF density with a fluid-fluid level
(D) multifocal attenuation of cortical tissue
(E) bilateral sickle-shaped densities over the hemispheres

---

123. Before 1930, men working as painters on ships developed wristdrops as a consequence of poisoning with

(A) mercury
(B) lead
(C) cadmium
(D) copper
(E) zinc

Traumatic and Occupational Injuries

Answers

112. The answer is B. *(Adams, ed 4. p 1068.)* Pressure on the volar aspect of the wrist may produce recurrent injuries to the carpal tunnel through which the median nerve runs. The injury characteristically produces pain and paresthesias in the hand over the distribution of the sensory component of the median nerve. This sensory distribution extends over the palmar surface of the thumb and first four digits, with the fourth digit supplied on one side by the median nerve and on the other side by the ulnar nerve. Median nerve injuries are consequently said to split the fourth digit on sensory examinations. With carpal tunnel compression of the median nerve, the sensory disturbance may be incapacitating. Subsequently, weakness and atrophy may develop in the muscles innervated by the median nerve. The abductor pollicis brevis may be severely involved late in the progression of the disorder.

113. The answer is A. *(Adams, ed 4. pp 1068–1069.)* Trauma to nerves in the extremities may give rise to causalgia, a disturbance in sensory perception characterized by hypesthesia, dysesthesia, and allodynia. Hypesthesia is a decrease in the accurate perception of stimuli. Dysesthesia is persistent discomfort, which in the situation described is likely to be an unremitting, burning pain. Allodynia is the perception of pain with the application of nonpainful stimuli. Bullets and other high-velocity missiles need not hit the nerve to cause damage. Enough energy is transmitted as the missile passes through adjacent tissues to produce substantial damage to the nerve.

114. The answer is C. *(Adams, ed 4. p 1068.)* The ulnar nerve runs superficially at the elbow in the ulnar groove. It continues forward under the aponeurosis of the flexor carpi ulnaris in the cubital tunnel. Damage to the nerve at this site may produce weakness in the interosseous and ulnar lumbrical muscles of the hand. With lumbrical weakness, the extensor sheaths of the digits are not properly positioned and a claw deformity with impaired extension of the ulnar two digits develops when the patient tries to straighten his or her fingers.

115. The answer is B. *(Lechtenberg, Synopsis, pp 127–128.)* Acoustic trauma may produce severe tinnitus in persons who have relatively little hearing loss. Although the initial injury with acoustic trauma is sustained by the cochlear sensory cells, tinnitus may persist even after the acoustic nerve is cut. Tinnitus may take any one of several forms, ranging from a hissing sound to a high-pitched screaming noise.

116. The answer is C. *(Adams, ed 4. p 1067.)* The musculocutaneous nerve is often damaged with fractures of the humerus. This nerve supplies the biceps brachii, brachialis, and coracobrachialis muscles and carries sensory information from the lateral cutaneous nerve of the forearm. Flexion at the elbow with damage to this nerve is most impaired with the forearm supinated.

117. The answer is D. *(Adams, ed 4. p 1067.)* Radial nerve injuries are fairly common in alcoholic persons who may have lost consciousness in awkward positions. These are sometimes referred to as "Saturday night palsies." The injury is usually a pressure palsy and produces a wristdrop. The nerve is injured as it courses near the spiral groove of the humerus.

118. The answer is A. *(Lechtenberg, Synopsis, pp 15–17.)* Within a few days of collection, the contents of the subdural hematoma are degraded into less-dense fluid. This fluid is transiently similar in density to the cerebral cortex. If the fluid collection is too small to produce substantial deformation of the underlying hemisphere, identification of the subdural collection may be difficult. An angiogram will reveal displacement of the cerebrocortical vessels, but more rapid and less invasive assessment of the patient is feasible with MR scanning.

119. The answer is C. *(Lechtenberg, Synopsis, pp 56–57.)* Something has abruptly caused increasing intracranial pressure in this young man after his head trauma. Consequently, he is at risk for herniation of the brain transfalcially or transtentorially, that is across the falx cerebri or across the tentorium cerebelli. The head trauma produced an intracranial lesion, which is expanding very rapidly. The slowing of his pulse and increase in his blood pressure is the Cushing effect of a rapidly expanding intracranial mass.

120. The answer is A. *(Adams, ed 4. p 704.)* Without emergency surgery this young man will die. His blood pressure and pulse abnormalities will correct themselves when the intracranial mass is removed. His loss of consciousness will not correct itself with antiepileptics. Shunt placement will not prevent brain herniation and may in fact accelerate it. The hematoma must be evacuated, and the bleeding giving rise to the hematoma must be stopped.

121. The answer is E. *(Adams, ed 4. p 704. Lechtenberg, Synopsis, pp 56–57.)* Damage to the middle meningeal artery allows blood at arterial pressures to dissect in the potential space that exists between the dura mater and the periosteum of the skull. Subarachnoid hemorrhage may have occurred along with the epidural bleeding, but the small amount of blood present in the CSF would be difficult to identify on MR scanning. With MR scanning the epidural hematoma should be evident soon after the injury and will certainly be evident by the time the patient is symptomatic.

122. The answer is B. *(Adams, ed 4. pp 704–705.)* The typical shape of an epidural hematoma is that of a biconvex mass displacing normal brain tissue. Parts of the ventricular system may be dilated as obstructive hydrocephalus develops in parts of the system. Transfalcial herniation with displacement of frontal lobe tissue across the midline and under the falx cerebri is likely with an epidural hematoma on one side of the head. Although subdural hematomas are often bilateral, epidural hematomas are invariably unilateral.

123. The answer is B. *(Adams, ed 4. pp 910–912.)* Lead poisoning may cause a pure motor neuropathy in adults. Lead-based paints are still a common cause of lead poisoning for children living in housing with old coats of paint. Children exposed to excessive lead levels may develop irritability, retardation, or increased intracranial pressure.

Infections

DIRECTIONS: Each question below contains five suggested responses. Select the **one best** response to each question.

124. All the following commonly produce microcephaly as a consequence of prenatal infection EXCEPT

(A) cytomegalovirus
(B) kuru
(C) toxoplasmosis
(D) rubella
(E) herpes simplex

125. Transmission of the type 1 human immunodeficiency virus (HIV-1) between humans has been well documented with all the following EXCEPT

(A) organ transplantation
(B) plasma exchange procedures
(C) packed red blood cell transfusions
(D) uncooked meal preparation
(E) artificial insemination

126. Sydenham chorea is a reversible chorea that develops as a consequence of

(A) hereditary degeneration of the caudate
(B) rheumatic fever
(C) posttraumatic degeneration of the substantia nigra
(D) subacute bacterial endocarditis
(E) Binswanger disease

127. Sydenham chorea develops most commonly in

(A) newborns
(B) boys between the ages of 3 and 7
(C) adolescent boys
(D) girls between the ages of 7 and 12
(E) adult women

128. The motor neuron disease most certainly traced to a virus is

(A) poliomyelitis
(B) subacute sclerosing panencephalitis (SSPE)
(C) progressive multifocal leukoencephalopathy (PML)
(D) subacute HIV encephalomyelitis
(E) kuru

129. The most common cause of cerebral mycosis, a fungal infection, is

(A) *Aspergillus*
(B) *Candida*
(C) *Mucor*
(D) *Cryptococcus*
(E) *Rhizopus*

130. *Schistosoma mansoni* ova usually damage the nervous system at the level of the

(A) cerebrum
(B) cerebellum
(C) basal ganglia
(D) spinal cord
(E) peripheral nerves

131. *Schistosoma japonicum* is primarily responsible for

(A) an encephalitis
(B) a mononeuritis multiplex
(C) a myelitis
(D) an encephalomyelitis
(E) a symmetric distal sensory neuropathy

132. Organs typically involved in cysticercosis include all the following EXCEPT

(A) brain
(B) muscle
(C) bladder
(D) eyes
(E) liver

133. The parasitic brain lesion most likely to have a large cyst containing numerous daughter cysts is that associated with

(A) *Taenia solium*
(B) *Schistosoma haematobium*
(C) *Taenia echinococcus*
(D) *Diphyllobothrium latum*
(E) *Schistosoma japonicum*

134. Acute and lethal malarial encephalitis is usually caused by

(A) none of the malarial organisms
(B) *Plasmodium vivax*
(C) *Plasmodium malariae*
(D) combined *Plasmodium vivax* and *P. malariae* infection
(E) *Plasmodium falciparum*

135. Cerebral amebic abscess is usually associated with concurrent disease in the

(A) eye
(B) spleen
(C) liver
(D) kidney
(E) spinal cord

136. Primary amebic meningoencephalitis is usually acquired through

(A) freshwater swimming
(B) eating contaminated meat
(C) eating calves' brains
(D) anal intercourse
(E) animal bites

137. What percentage of patients with the inflammatory disease sarcoidosis have symptomatic neurologic disease?

(A) 1 percent
(B) 5 percent
(C) 20 percent
(D) 50 percent
(E) 80 percent

138. The cranial nerve most often injured in sarcoidosis is

(A) II
(B) III
(C) V
(D) VII
(E) VIII

139. The peripheral neuropathy associated with sarcoidosis commonly presents as

(A) mononeuritis multiplex
(B) brachial plexitis
(C) pure motor neuropathy
(D) dysautonomia
(E) lumbosacral plexopathy

140. All the following are highly probable with neurosarcoidosis EXCEPT

(A) hydrocephalus
(B) intracranial vasculopathy
(C) seizures
(D) hypothalamic granuloma
(E) cerebellar atrophy

141. All the following signs and symptoms are probable with neurosarcoidosis EXCEPT

(A) fever
(B) leukocytosis with eosinophilia
(C) positive skin-tuberculin reaction
(D) uveitis
(E) elevated serum levels of angiotensin converting enzyme

142. The 6-month-old child who develops a febrile seizure should be investigated with a spinal tap because

(A) all febrile seizures justify spinal taps
(B) most febrile seizures are from bacterial infections
(C) febrile seizures cause increased intracranial pressure, which must be relieved by withdrawing CSF
(D) intrathecal antiepileptics must be given
(E) children this age may have meningitis with no manifestations other than fever and seizures

143. With simple febrile convulsions, the most likely seizure type is a

(A) complex partial seizure
(B) generalized tonic-clonic seizure
(C) generalized absence seizure
(D) focal motor seizure
(E) focal sensory seizure

144. All the following are associated with an infection caused by *Corynebacterium diphtheriae* EXCEPT

(A) polyneuropathy
(B) impaired visual accommodation
(C) aphonia
(D) myocarditis
(E) nephritis

145. Neurologic signs and symptoms of tuberculous meningitis include all the following EXCEPT

(A) headache
(B) diplopia
(C) vomiting
(D) seizures
(E) confabulation

146. Mass lesions in the brain of the patient with tuberculosis may develop as a reaction to the tubercle bacillus and consist of

(A) dysplastic CNS tissue
(B) caseating granulomas
(C) heterotopias
(D) colobomas
(E) mesial sclerosis

147. The CSF changes seen with tuberculous meningitis are very much like those associated with

(A) a fungal meningitis
(B) a slow viral encephalitis
(C) a brain abscess
(D) cysticercosis
(E) subarachnoid hemorrhage

148. Confirmation of the diagnosis of tuberculous meningitis proves impossible in what percentage of patients?

(A) 0
(B) 5 percent
(C) 15 percent
(D) 30 percent
(E) 50 percent

149. Antibiotic treatment of tuberculous meningitis should include

(A) 1 year of isoniazid and chloramphenicol
(B) 9 months of isoniazid and rifampin
(C) 2 years of isoniazid and rifampin
(D) 6 months of ethambutol and rifampin
(E) 18 months of ethambutol and rifampin

150. All the following are predisposing factors for meningitis with *Streptococcus pneumoniae* EXCEPT

(A) CSF leaks
(B) acute sinusitis
(C) epilepsy
(D) acute otitis media
(E) sickle cell anemia

151. Persons exposed to a patient with meningococcal meningitis should receive prophylactic

(A) rifampin
(B) isoniazid
(C) penicillin G
(D) tetracycline
(E) ethambutol

152. Gram-negative bacillary meningitis usually develops in

(A) neonates
(B) infants 6 months to 2 years of age
(C) infants 2 to 4 years of age
(D) children 4 to 12 years of age
(E) adolescents

153. The drug of choice with *Listeria monocytogenes* meningitis is

(A) penicillin G
(B) ampicillin
(C) tetracycline
(D) gentamicin
(E) rifampin

154. Recurrent meningitis often develops in persons with

(A) otitis media
(B) epilepsy
(C) multiple sclerosis
(D) Whipple's disease
(E) CSF leaks

155. Localization of an encephalitis to the medial temporal or orbital frontal regions of the brain is most consistent with

(A) *Treponema pallidum*
(B) varicella zoster
(C) herpes simplex
(D) *Cryptococcus neoformans*
(E) *Toxoplasma gondii*

156. Neuroimaging of the brain before attempting a lumbar puncture is advisable in cases of herpes encephalitis because

(A) the diagnosis may be evident on the basis of MR scanning alone
(B) massive edema in the temporal lobe may make herniation imminent
(C) the CT picture may determine whether a brain biopsy should be obtained
(D) shunting of the ventricles is usually indicated and the imaging studies are needed to direct the placement of the shunt
(E) it may establish whether type 1 or type 2 is responsible

157. The CSF changes late in the course of herpes encephalitis typically include

(A) an increased number of mononuclear cells
(B) a glucose content of less than two-thirds the serum level
(C) a protein content of less than 45 mg/dL
(D) a normal opening pressure
(E) a predominance of polymorphonuclear white blood cells

158. With herpes encephalitis the EEG may exhibit

(A) alpha activity over the frontal regions
(B) beta activity over the temporal regions
(C) three per second spike-and-wave discharges
(D) bilateral, periodic epileptiform discharges
(E) unilateral delta activity over the frontal region

159. Once the diagnosis of herpes encephalitis has been reached, the most appropriate treatment is

(A) cyclophosphamide
(B) amphotericin B
(C) gamma globulin
(D) methotrexate
(E) acyclovir

160. The pathologic feature most likely to be seen in the brain with subacute HIV encephalomyelitis is the

(A) Lewy body
(B) Pick body
(C) neurofibrillary tangle
(D) astrocyte proliferation
(E) syncytial cell

161. Opportunistic infections commonly involving the CNS in patients with AIDS include

(A) pneumococcal meningitis
(B) cryptococcal meningitis
(C) meningococcal meningitis
(D) *Haemophilus influenzae* meningitis
(E) enterococcal meningitis

162. Contrast-enhanced intracranial lesions appearing as rings in the patient with AIDS are likely to indicate

(A) *Listeria monocytogenes* abscesses
(B) streptococcal abscesses
(C) multifocal meningiomas
(D) *Treponema pallidum* granulomas
(E) *Toxoplasma* granulomas

163. The neoplasm most likely to develop in the brain of the HIV-infected person is

(A) Kaposi's sarcoma
(B) oligodendroglioma
(C) glioblastoma multiforme
(D) primary lymphoma
(E) meningioma

164. HIV appears to enter the CNS in persons who eventually develop subacute HIV encephalomyelitis by

(A) the infiltration of free viral particles across the blood-brain barrier
(B) the migration of infected macrophages into the CNS
(C) acquisition of the virus by ependymal cells from contaminated CSF
(D) migration of the virus proximally along nerve fibers
(E) subclinical subarachnoid hemorrhages

165. Progressive multifocal leukoencephalopathy (PML) may develop in the patient with AIDS as a consequence of

(A) papovavirus infection
(B) HIV-1 infection
(C) herpesvirus infection
(D) zidovudine (AZT) therapy
(E) amphotericin B therapy

166. Seizures may develop in the patient with AIDS as a consequence of any of the following EXCEPT

(A) progressive multifocal leukoencephalopathy (PML)
(B) nocardial brain abscesses
(C) herpes encephalitis
(D) mycobacterial meningoencephalitis
(E) zidovudine (AZT) toxicity

167. All the following usually develop with Reye syndrome EXCEPT

(A) hyperglycemia
(B) cerebral edema
(C) fatty vacuolization of the renal tubules
(D) fatty vacuolization of the liver
(E) neuronal degeneration in the brain

168. One of the medications often implicated in children with Reye syndrome is

(A) tetracycline
(B) penicillin G
(C) ceftriaxone
(D) acetaminophen
(E) aspirin

169. Both HIV and cytomegalovirus infections in the brain characteristically produce

(A) senile plaques
(B) intraneuronal amyloid
(C) intranuclear inclusions
(D) intracytoplasmic inclusions
(E) microglial nodules

170. With congenital rubella infection, the child may exhibit all the following EXCEPT

(A) cataracts
(B) pigmentary retinopathy
(C) glaucoma
(D) saber shins
(E) structural heart lesions

171. Any of the following may produce the constellation of congenital rash, jaundice, hepatomegaly, retinitis, splenomegaly, cataracts, and microcephaly EXCEPT

(A) rubella
(B) *Listeria monocytogenes*
(C) cytomegalovirus
(D) herpes simplex
(E) *Toxoplasma gondii*

172. *Borrelia burgdorferi* infection is likely to produce all the following EXCEPT

(A) rash
(B) meningoencephalitis
(C) hepatitis
(D) arthritis
(E) myocarditis

173. After *B. burgdorferi* is introduced by the tick that carries it, the skin around the bite develops

(A) an exfoliative dermatitis
(B) purpura
(C) localized edema
(D) erythema chronicum migrans
(E) vesicular lesions

174. False positive tests for Lyme disease may develop if the patient has

(A) rheumatoid arthritis
(B) subacute bacterial endocarditis
(C) scleroderma
(D) syphilis
(E) dermatomyositis

175. The cranial neuropathy most commonly associated with Lyme disease is that associated with damage to cranial nerve

(A) III
(B) V
(C) VII
(D) IX
(E) XII

176. Early in its evolution, neurologic abnormalities caused by Lyme disease include all the following EXCEPT

(A) cerebrocortical atrophy
(B) acute transverse myelitis
(C) lumbar plexitis
(D) aseptic meningitis
(E) demyelinating polyneuritis

177. The medication most appropriate in patients with CNS involvement by *Borrelia burgdorferi* is

(A) streptomycin
(B) ceftriaxone
(C) gentamicin
(D) isoniazid
(E) rifampin

178. Abscesses in the brain most often develop from

(A) hematogenous spread of infection
(B) penetrating head wounds
(C) superinfection of neoplastic foci
(D) dental trauma
(E) neurosurgical intervention

179. The most common site for abscess formation in the brain is

(A) in the putamen
(B) in the thalamus
(C) in the head of the caudate
(D) at the gray-white junction
(E) in the subthalamus

180. Most of the organisms found in brain abscesses are

(A) streptococcal
(B) staphylococcal
(C) *Bacteroides* species
(D) *Proteus* species
(E) *Pseudomonas* species

181. The most common cause of brain abscess in the patient with AIDS is

(A) *Cryptococcus neoformans*
(B) *Toxoplasma gondii*
(C) tuberculosis
(D) cytomegalovirus
(E) herpes zoster

182. The most common complaint in the patient with brain abscess is

(A) nausea and vomiting
(B) ataxia
(C) headache
(D) neck stiffness
(E) seizures

183. The diagnostic test most likely to reveal a brain abscess is

(A) CT scan
(B) MR scan
(C) pneumoencephalogram
(D) arteriogram
(E) radionuclide brain scan

184. Fungal abscesses in the brain are most commonly caused by

(A) *Nocardia*
(B) *Cryptococcus neoformans*
(C) *Actinomyces*
(D) *Aspergillus*
(E) *Candida*

185. All the following typically develop with tabes dorsalis EXCEPT

(A) personality changes
(B) lancinating pains
(C) ataxia
(D) impaired position sense
(E) impaired pupillary reflexes

186. Neurosyphilis may present a picture easily confused with brain tumor if

(A) a reaction to penicillin treatment occurs
(B) an intracranial gumma forms
(C) tabes dorsalis is the primary manifestation of the disease
(D) meningovascular syphilis develops
(E) the patient is a newborn with congenital syphilis

187. General paresis is a form of neurosyphilis caused by

(A) a response to penicillin treatment
(B) an autoimmune reaction
(C) an acute meningoencephalitis
(D) a chronic meningoencephalitis
(E) a chronic rhombencephalitis

188. Which of the following viruses typically invades the CNS by extending centripetally along peripheral nerves?

(A) Mumps
(B) Measles
(C) Varicella zoster
(D) Poliovirus
(E) Rabies

189. From the brain, the rabies virus establishes itself for transmission to another host by spreading to the

(A) intestines
(B) nasopharynx
(C) lungs
(D) bladder
(E) salivary glands

190. Hydrophobia develops in many patients with rabies as a manifestation of

(A) dysesthesias in the mouth on exposure to water
(B) an anaphylactic reaction to water
(C) a delusional reaction to fluids
(D) spasmotic contractions of respiratory muscles on attempts at drinking
(E) opisthotonus triggered by attempts at drinking

191. The best therapy currently available for rabies is

(A) supportive therapy
(B) zidovudine
(C) cytarabine
(D) amantadine
(E) ganciclovir

192. With Creutzfeldt-Jakob disease the EEG will usually evolve as the patient deteriorates to a pattern characterized by

(A) three per second spike-and-wave activity
(B) focal slowing to 3 to 5 Hz over the parietal lobes
(C) disorganized background activity with repetitive discharges at approximately one per second
(D) prominent triphasic waves most evident over the frontal leads
(E) electrocerebral silence

193. All the following are consistent with Guillain-Barré syndrome EXCEPT

(A) 5-day history of progressive weakness
(B) antecedent infection of upper respiratory tract
(C) absent deep tendon reflexes
(D) impaired pain perception below T4 dermatome
(E) flexor plantar responses

194. The test most likely to establish the diagnosis of Guillain-Barré syndrome is

(A) examination of CSF
(B) visual evoked potential
(C) somatosensory evoked potential
(D) brainstem auditory evoked potential
(E) routine electroencephalography

195. The skeletal muscles usually spared with Guillain-Barré syndrome are

(A) diaphragmatic
(B) oculomotor
(C) interosseous
(D) interphalangeal
(E) oropharyngeal

Infections

Answers

124. The answer is B. *(Davis, p 225.)* These congenital infections producing microcephaly are included in the TORCH group. Kuru also causes encephalitis, but it is acquired in childhood or adult life after brain formation has been completed. Kuru is a slow viral infection that occurs in the Fore Islanders of New Guinea. It is pathologically similar to Creutzfeldt-Jakob disease, another slow viral illness that produces tremor, ataxia, dementia, and inanition and is found in the U.S. and other industrialized nations. Microcephaly may also develop as a consequence of metabolic diseases, such as phenylketonuria and Tay-Sachs disease. Tay-Sachs more commonly produces macrocephaly, but finding microcephaly does not eliminate the diagnosis.

125. The answer is D. *(Lechtenberg, AIDS, pp 26–30.)* All modes of HIV-1 transmission are probably not yet known, but transmission of the virus through food has yet to be suggested by patterns of disease spread. The virus is sensitive to heat and other environmental stresses, and so it should not survive in most cooked materials. Ingestion of infected material may transmit the virus, although the viability of the virus in the face of gastric acids is likely to be poor. Fellatio is nonetheless a suspected mode of transmission for the virus.

126. The answer is B. *(Lechtenberg, Synopsis, p 86.)* Most choreas are transient phenomena associated with viral or bacterial infections. Sydenham chorea develops with a group A streptococcal infection. It is a primary feature of rheumatic fever along with arthritis and endocarditis. Degeneration of the caudate nucleus occurs in the hereditary form of chorea called Huntington disease. Trauma to the basal ganglia may produce parkinsonism but does not typically produce chorea. Subacute bacterial endocarditis is a cardiac disease that, like rheumatic fever, may produce damage to the heart valves, but it is not associated with a movement disorder. Binswanger disease is a vascular disease that may cause widespread cerebral damage, but dementia, rather than chorea, is the most prominent consequence of this disease.

127. The answer is D. *(Lechtenberg, Synopsis, p 86.)* Sydenham chorea may recur years after the acute episode has completely remitted. It will usually reappear on exposure to hormones, such as those in birth control pills, or during pregnancy. Some persons develop recurrent movements if they take phenytoin. The initial episode of Sydenham chorea requires no treatment. It is invariably self-limited. Using phenothiazines or butyrophenones to suppress the transient chorea exposes the child to the risk of other movement disorders, such as tardive dyskinesia.

128. The answer is A. *(Lechtenberg, Synopsis, p 100.)* SSPE, PML, kuru, and HIV encephalomyelitis are all viral diseases affecting the CNS, but poliomyelitis is the only one that causes a purely motor neuron disease. Poliomyelitis virus attacks the anterior horn cells in the spinal cord. It is most likely to be confused with Guillain-Barré syndrome if the typical CSF picture of a viral meningoencephalitis is not found with the progressive motor neuron impairment. With poliomyelitis, the CSF will usually exhibit an elevated protein and white cell count. During the initial stages of the infection, the patient will usually have fever.

129. The answer is D. *(Davis, pp 667–668.)* Cryptococcosis is usually acquired through the lungs. It spreads to the CNS through the bloodstream. In the CNS, it may produce either a meningitis or a meningoencephalitis. The organism has a characteristic capsule, which simplifies its identification. Fungal infections most often occur in the CNS in persons with defects in their immune systems. These defects may be secondary to a viral infection, as is the case with AIDS, or they may be a consequence of immunosuppressive drug exposure. Patients who were on immunosuppressive treatment after organ transplants and who had lymphoproliferative disorders, such as lymphocytic leukemia, were the most common victims of CNS fungal infections before the start of the AIDS epidemic.

130. The answer is D. *(Davis, pp 693–694.)* *Schistosoma mansoni* is endemic in Puerto Rico and may produce a subacutely evolving paraparesis. The fluke itself does not invade the spinal cord, but it deposits eggs in the valveless veins of Batson, which drain the intestines and communicate with the drainage from the lumbosacral spinal cord. The patient develops granulomas around the ova that lodge in the spinal cord, and these granulomatous lesions crush the cord.

131. The answer is A. *(Davis, pp 693–694.)* The ova of *S. japonicum* are small and the spine on the surface of the ovum is small in comparison with that occurring with *S. mansoni* and *S. haematobium*. This allows the ova to embolize to the brain where they produce an inflammatory response characterized by multinucleated giant cells, reactive astrocytes, and chronic lymphocytic infiltration. This encephalitis may appear weeks or months after exposure to the parasite and is often fatal.

132. The answer is C. *(Davis, pp 687–689.)* Cysticercosis is produced by the pork tapeworm, *Taenia solium.* This is transmitted through infected human feces to animals and usually through infected pork to man. This is still a common parasitic disease in Mexico, the Philippines, and India. Cysticercal infection of muscles produces a nonspecific myositis. Brain involvement may lead to seizures. The lesions in the brain may calcify and often appear as multiple small cysts spread throughout the cerebrum.

133. The answer is C. *(Davis, pp 689–690.)* Echinococcosis is usually acquired by eating tissue from infected sheep. Children are more likely to develop cerebral lesions than adults, but people at any age may develop this encephalic hydatidosis, which entails the development of a major cyst with multiple compartments in which smaller cysts are evident. This hydatid cyst of the brain behaves like a tumor and may become massive enough to cause focal deficits.

134. The answer is E. *(Davis, p 679.)* Falciparum malaria is transmitted by the *Anopheles* mosquito. It is still the most important parasitic disease of man and accounts for about 1 million deaths worldwide annually. Children with no immunity to malaria are most likely to develop the cerebral form. Persons with sickle cell trait or sickle cell disease have slight resistance to the parasite.

135. The answer is C. *(Davis, p 678.)* Cerebral amebiasis is caused by *Entamoeba histolytica* and is still fairly common in Mexico. It is carried to the CNS through the bloodstream. The organism gains a foothold initially in the intestines before spreading to the liver and the lungs. Abscesses in the brain usually develop at the gray-white junctions of the cerebral hemispheres.

136. The answer is A. *(Davis, pp 676–678.)* Primary amebic meningoencephalitis is usually caused by organisms from the genera *Hartmanella* or *Acanthamoeba.* The parasites enter the nervous system through the cribriform plate at the perforations for the olfactory nerves. An especially lethal form of this meningoencephalitis may develop with *Naegleria* species. Other parasites, such as *Schistosoma mansoni,* may be acquired through swimming in contaminated freshwater, but it is unlikely that other parasites reach the nervous system through direct invasion across the cribriform plate. Schistosomiasis is acquired when the cercarial phase of the organism penetrates the swimmer's skin and finds its way into the blood.

137. The answer is B. *(Johnson, ed 3. p 154.)* Sarcoid produces noncaseating granulomas in a variety of organs, including the lungs, liver, spleen, and skin. Its evolution may be fulminant or exceedingly slow. CNS involvement ranges from retinal disease to aseptic meningitis. The lesions most likely in the central nervous system include noncaseating granulomas, transverse myelitis, optic neuritis, and aseptic meningitis.

138. The answer is D. *(Johnson, ed 3. p 154.)* Facial paresis is the neurologic injury most likely to develop with sarcoidosis. Almost half the patients with sarcoidosis and neurologic disease have a neurologic sign or symptom as the first obvious complication of the sarcoidosis. The patients report progressive weakness of one side of the face with no substantial loss of sensation over the paretic side. They may feel that there is decreased sensitivity to touch on the weak side, but this is more commonly from a loss of tone in the facial muscles than from an injury to the trigeminal nerve. Other cranial nerves especially susceptible to injury in persons with sarcoidosis include II, III, IV, VI, and VIII.

139. The answer is A. *(Rowland, ed 8. pp 149–151.)* A symmetric distal sensory neuropathy is also a fairly common complication of neurosarcoidosis. With mononeuritis multiplex, the most common peripheral nerve problem with sarcoidosis, an individual nerve is damaged and focal deficits appear in the muscles and skin supplied by that nerve. Although recovery from the individual nerve injury is likely over the course of weeks or months, other nerves will be disabled as lesions skip from one nerve to another.

140. The answer is E. *(Rowland, ed 8. pp 149–151.)* Meningitis or meningoencephalitis may develop with neurosarcoidosis, but the cerebellum is not a specific target and cerebellar atrophy should not be ascribed to sarcoidosis. A chronic adhesive arachnoiditis frequently develops with the aseptic meningitis of sarcoidosis, and the posterior fossa is an especially common location for this arachnoiditis. Large parenchymal lesions, such as granulomas and infarctions, may develop in the cerebellum, as well as in the cerebrum, but such injuries are relatively rare.

141. The answer is C. *(Rowland, ed 8. pp 149–151.)* Patients with sarcoid are often anergic, and so their skin tests are likely to be negative even if they have been exposed to tuberculosis. Many patients have a chronic anemia and hypercalcemia. Serum levels of gamma globulin are elevated in about half the patients affected.

142. The answer is E. *(Johnson, ed 3. p 30.)* Between birth and 1 year of age, what appears to be a simple febrile seizure may actually be a seizure provoked by a bacterial meningitis. The agents most likely to be responsible are *Haemophilus influenzae* and *Enterococcus coli*. Both require rapid diagnosis and early treatment if the child is to survive. *E. coli* is unlikely after the newborn period. Both infections require CSF examination for the diagnosis.

143. The answer is B. *(Johnson, ed 3. pp 29–30.)* Simple febrile seizures last less than 15 min and have no focal characteristics. The child has no persistent neurologic deficits after the seizure, and multiple seizures do not typically occur during any individual febrile episode. These seizures occur during childhood and are most likely between 1 and 5 years of age. They produce no apparent brain damage and do not increase the probability that the child will have epilepsy later in life.

144. The answer is E. *(Adams, ed 4. pp 908–909.)* Diphtherial infection may produce a variety of neurologic signs and symptoms. Local pharyngeal involvement and cranial nerve injury may produce aphonia and dysphagia. Paralysis of accommodation is an additional component of the polyneuropathy that is similar to that occurring with botulism. It usually develops days or weeks after palatal dysfunction. Cardiac muscle involvement is another manifestation of remote effects of an exotoxin produced by the bacterium. Patients may die from respiratory failure associated with the neuropathy or from cardiac failure associated with the cardiomyopathy.

145. The answer is E. *(Johnson, ed 3. p 134.)* Dementia may develop as a complication of tuberculous meningitis, but the confabulation typical of the memory disturbance seen with chronic alcoholism is not at all likely with tuberculous meningitis. Patients develop diplopia because third, fourth, and sixth cranial palsies may appear with granulomatous inflammation about the arteries at the base of the skull. With long-standing inflammation about the vessels, thromboses may develop within the vessels.

146. The answer is B. *(Johnson, ed 3. pp 134–135.)* Rupture of a large caseating granuloma into the ventricles or the subarachnoid space may produce an abrupt and often lethal deterioration. If the mass becomes large enough before it ruptures, it may in all respects imitate a brain tumor. Such lesions may respond to antituberculous medications even when they are quite large, and the patient may be spared surgical intervention.

147. The answer is A. *(Johnson, ed 3. pp 134–135.)* Typically the CSF in both tuberculous and fungal meningitis exhibits a high protein, a low or moderately low glucose content, and an increase in mononuclear white blood cells. With both types of meningitis, an extraordinary range of CSF changes is seen. If a granuloma acutely ruptures, the CSF with tuberculous meningitis may have a high number of polymorphonuclear cells but convert to a mononuclear pattern over the course of days.

148. The answer is C. *(Johnson, ed 3. pp 134–135.)* Only about one-third of the CSF smears from patients with tuberculous meningitis will reveal tubercle bacilli. Only one-half of the cultures performed on CSF in infected patients will grow the tubercle bacilli. Because so large a part of the general population has been exposed to the tubercle bacillus and so many of them have positive skin tests for years before the appearance of an acute or chronic meningitis, many patients are treated for tuberculous meningitis on the basis of very scanty evidence.

149. The answer is B. *(Johnson, ed 3. pp 135–136.)* Many physicians still use triple therapy with isoniazid, rifampin, and ethambutol to treat tuberculous meningitis, but this has no distinct advantages over therapy with just two drugs. If the antibiotic regimen is intended to be briefer than 9 months, then management with ethambutol or streptomycin or pyrazinamide or two of these agents in combination with isoniazid and rifampin may be appropriate. The reason such four-drug regimens are usually not adopted is that the combined toxicity of these drugs is unacceptably high in most patients.

150. The answer is C. *(Johnson, ed 3. p 132.)* Pneumococcal meningitis may also develop in association with pneumonia caused by this organism or in a patient who has an impaired immune system. Patients with AIDS do not have a substantial increase in streptococcal meningitis, even though the level of meningoencephalitis occurring with AIDS is greatly increased. Penicillin G is still the drug of choice for treating pneumococcal pneumonia.

151. The answer is A. *(Johnson, ed 3. p 132.)* Meningococcal meningitis is caused by *Neisseria meningitidis*. It occurs episodically or epidemically, and usually affects young adults. Once the meningitis has been established, penicillin G is the drug of choice.

152. The answer is A. *(Johnson, ed 3. pp 132–133.)* Gram-negative bacillary meningitis may develop in immunocompromised persons after the newborn period, but it is relatively rare in any age group. Patients occasionally contract this type of infection after head trauma or neurosurgical procedures. The drug of choice for an *E. coli* meningitis is a combination of ceftriaxone and gentamicin.

153. The answer is B. *(Johnson, ed 3. pp 132–133.)* *L. monocytogenes* meningitis develops in renal transplant recipients, patients with chronic renal disease, immunosuppressed persons, and occasionally in otherwise unimpaired persons. It may on occasion lead to intracerebral abscess formation. This type of meningitis is not usually seen in infants or children.

154. The answer is E. *(Johnson, ed 3. pp 133–134.)* A CSF leak indicates a communication between the subarachnoid space and the surface of the body. This leak most often occurs through the nose as rhinorrhea or through the ear as otorrhea. CSF may be distinguished from other fluid discharged from the nose or ear by its relatively obvious glucose content. The most common basis for a CSF leak is head trauma.

155. The answer is C. *(Johnson, ed 3. p 116.)* Herpes simplex type 1 is the strain usually responsible for a herpetic encephalitis. Type 2 may occur in newborns who have been exposed during their passage through the birth canal of a woman with genital herpes. Persons with AIDS are also at risk for either type 1 or type 2. Temporal lobe involvement in the immunocompetent patient may produce unilateral swelling and hemorrhage into the temporal lobe.

156. The answer is B. *(Johnson, ed 3. p 116.)* Although there is some controversy regarding whether or not lumbar puncture can precipitate herniation with a herpes encephalitis, most authorities believe it is best to assess the risk of herniation before doing a lumbar puncture. CSF examination is vital in establishing the diagnosis. A variety of infections may mimic herpes in both its course and anatomic distribution. CSF cultures and analysis of CSF constituents help to establish the probable cause of the encephalitis and to direct therapy.

157. The answer is A. *(Johnson, ed 3. pp 116–117.)* The increased number of mononuclear cells in the CSF of the patient with herpes encephalitis ranges from more than a dozen to several hundred mononuclear cells per cubic millimeter of fluid. Red blood cells may be apparent in the CSF late in the course of the disease, but their absence does not eliminate the possibility of herpes encephalitis. CSF pressure is usually increased and the glucose content is usually normal or only slightly depressed.

158. The answer is D. *(Johnson, ed 3. pp 116–117.)* The periodic discharges seen with herpes encephalitis typically occur over the temporal regions. Slow waves, rather than sharp waves, may be evident over the temporal lobes in many persons with severe disease. Seizures commonly occur early in the course of herpes encephalitis, and so the EEG may be severely disturbed generally.

159. The answer is E. *(Johnson, ed 3. p 117.)* The diagnosis of herpes encephalitis is more controversial than the treatment. Many authorities believe brain biopsy should be performed whenever the diagnosis is suspected, but most believe that a normal CSF glucose in association with the typical features of a herpes encephalitis should be sufficient grounds for starting acyclovir treatment. The acyclovir must be given intravenously for 10 days.

160. The answer is E. *(Lechtenberg, AIDS, pp 44–47.)* The syncytial cell is a diseased macrophage that has fused with other macrophages and has a typical multinuclear configuration. The brain injured by HIV infection usually has many of these cells and many microglial nodules. Myelin pallor is also evident in widely scattered regions of the brain and spinal cord.

161. The answer is B. *(Lechtenberg, AIDS, pp 80–83.)* Fungal infections are common problems inside and outside the CNS in patients with AIDS. Treatment for cryptococcal meningitis in these patients requires the use of amphotericin B, an extremely toxic antifungal agent. Even with uninterrupted antifungal treatment, patients with this opportunistic infection often die as a consequence of cryptococcal meningoencephalitis.

162. The answer is E. *(Lechtenberg, AIDS, pp 63–75.)* *Toxoplasma gondii* is an obligate intracellular parasite that produces cysts, pseudocysts, and granulomas in the brains of HIV-infected persons. Lesions are often multiple and widely scattered throughout the brain. They are easily visualized on CT and MR imaging.

163. The answer is D. *(Lechtenberg, AIDS, pp 99–104.)* Primary brain lymphomas were distinctly uncommon intracranial neoplasms until the advent of AIDS. The tumors may appear very similar to *Toxoplasma* granulomas on CT and MR scanning. Irradiation of the brain may be of value in managing the neoplasm, but survival of the affected patient has been poor regardless of the treatment attempted.

164. The answer is B. *(Lechtenberg, AIDS, pp 35–38.)* Macrophages infected with HIV may carry the virus into the CNS uneventfully, until something activates the virus in the infected cells. Whether another virus or just incidental macrophage activity is the key to activating the AIDS virus is unknown. A person with HIV infection may remain asymptomatic for months or years.

165. The answer is A. *(Lechtenberg, AIDS, pp 83–92.)* The papovavirus behaves like an opportunistic infection in the person with AIDS. Specific types of papovavirus likely to attack the CNS in these patients include BK, JC, and SV-40. The patient with the demyelinating disease PML caused by this papovavirus infection usually has deteriorating cognitive and motor function over the course of weeks or months.

166. The answer is E. *(Lechtenberg, AIDS, pp 123–135.)* Zidovudine (azidothymidine, AZT) may cause leukopenia or other types of marrow depression, but it does not have an irritative effect on the brain. Treatment with zidovudine does improve neurologic function in most persons with symptomatic CNS complications of AIDS, but that does not mean that this antiviral agent can halt or reverse CNS damage directly attributable to HIV. Current information suggests that minor neurologic deterioration occurs in patients on zidovudine who are otherwise stable in terms of their immunodeficiency state.

167. The answer is A. *(Wilson, ed 12. pp 1353–1354.)* Reye syndrome occurs in children 2 to 15 years of age. Patients with Reye syndrome usually develop hypoglycemia and require emergency infusions of glucose. Intravenous mannitol and fresh frozen plasma have also been used to reduce the cerebral edema and bleeding disorders characteristically seen with this disease. Only about half of the affected persons survive, and those who do usually exhibit liver damage.

168. The answer is E. *(Wilson, ed 12. pp 1353–1354.)* Although there has been much experience connecting salicylate use to the development of Reye syndrome, cases of this syndrome have occurred in children not exposed to aspirin or other salicylates. The upper respiratory tract infections with which this syndrome most commonly occurs are those caused by chickenpox or influenza viruses. Patients who die usually succumb to liver failure.

169. The answer is E. *(Lechtenberg, AIDS, pp 75–79.)* The microglial nodules occurring with HIV are associated with syncytial cells in the brain and spinal cord, a cell type not typically seen with cytomegalovirus (CMV) encephalitis. CMV is a common CNS opportunistic agent in patients with AIDS. With HIV infection, the microglial nodules are distributed around blood vessels throughout the brain. With CMV, the nodules are more characteristically subpial and subependymal.

170. The answer is D. *(Johnson, ed 3. p 111.)* Saber shins are typical of patients with congenital syphilis, not congenital rubella. The infant born with rubella may have widely disseminated disease that produces pneumonitis, hepatitis, cardiomyopathy, and encephalitis. Anemia, jaundice, and thrombocytopenia associated with congenital rubella are usually transient. Many children with intrauterine rubella will have sensorineural hearing loss and retardation.

171. The answer is B. *(Johnson, ed 3. p 111.)* The constellation described is the classic TORCH syndrome, a congenital syndrome usually associated with toxoplasmosis, rubella, cytomegalovirus, or herpes infection. *Listeria monocytogenes* may cause infection that attacks the pregnant uterus, but it most commonly produces recurrent miscarriages. Any infant surviving these congenital TORCH infections is likely to have hearing, motor, visual, and cognitive problems.

172. The answer is C. *(Adams, ed 4. pp 580–581.)* *Borrelia burgdorferi* is the agent responsible for Lyme disease. It is a spirochete usually transmitted to man through tick bites. Multiple organ systems are attacked by the spirochete, and the nervous system is especially susceptible.

173. The answer is D. *(Johnson, ed 3. p 148.)* Erythema chronicum migrans is an expanding reddish discoloration of the skin that spreads away from the site of the bite as an expanding ring of erythema. It usually evolves over 3 to 4 weeks. This ring of erythema clears spontaneously within about a month and is usually associated with some headache and neck stiffness. Some patients with Lyme disease fail to exhibit the rash.

174. The answer is D. *(Johnson, ed 3. p 148.)* Both Lyme disease and syphilis are caused by spirochetes. A false positive Lyme test may also occur with relapsing fever, but this is much less of a problem in the U.S. than in countries where relapsing fever is endemic. Tests for the Lyme antibody with the western blot technique are sensitive and specific and should be used when the diagnosis is suspected.

175. The answer is C. *(Adams, ed 4. pp 580–581.)* Facial weakness may be the only neurologic sign of Lyme disease. The neurologic deficits usually appear weeks after the initial rash. Untreated neurologic disease may persist for months. The facial palsy or optic neuritis that develops with CNS disease is characteristically associated with a meningitis.

176. The answer is A. *(Johnson, ed 3. pp 148–149.)* In Lyme disease, numerous sites inside and outside the CNS will be damaged, but the disease does not attack neurons early in its course. Late in the disease, a dementia similar to that seen in general paresis may develop, but that is rare and improbable if the patient has been treated with antibiotics. Additional neurologic problems include mononeuritis multiplex, focal encephalitis, and cerebral vasculitis.

177. The answer is B. *(Johnson, ed 3. pp 149–150.)* This organism is sensitive to cefotaxime and erythromycin, as well as to ceftriaxone. Amoxicillin or tetracycline is effective in many patients, but incomplete eradication of the organism is a common problem in patients not treated with the most specific antibiotics. If CNS complications do develop, the patient should receive intravenous penicillin or cefotaxime for at least 10 days.

178. The answer is A. *(Johnson, ed 3. p 136.)* There are many bases for abscess formation in the brain, but the most frequent causes are blood-borne infections from sources in the lung, heart, sinuses, and ears. Extension of infection from a chronic otitis or mastoiditis was much more common before the introduction of antibiotics. Facial or dental infections may spread to the brain through valveless veins draining about the muscles of mastication and communicating with the venous drainage of the brain.

179. The answer is D. *(Johnson, ed 3. p 137.)* The brain abscess usually starts from a microscopic focus of infection at the junction of gray matter and white matter. As the infection develops, a cerebritis appears, and subsequently this focus of infection becomes necrotic and liquefies. Around the enlarging abscess there is usually a large area of edema.

180. The answer is A. *(Johnson, ed 3. p 137.)* Both aerobic and anaerobic streptococcal bacteria occur in more than half of all brain abscesses. *Staphylococcus aureus* most often occurs in patients who have had penetrating head wounds or undergone neurosurgical procedures. Enteric bacteria, such as *E. coli, Proteus,* and *Pseudomonas,* account for twice as many abscesses as *S. aureus.*

181. The answer is B. *(Johnson, ed 3. p 137.)* Fungal abscesses develop with unusual frequency in patients with AIDS, but *T. gondii,* an obligate intracellular parasite, is considerably more common than fungi as the cause of abscess formation. The fungi that do produce abscesses in persons with AIDS are most often *Cryptococcus, Candida, Mucor,* and *Aspergillus.* Mycobacteria and atypical mycobacteria are also common causes of abscess formation in some populations.

182. The answer is C. *(Johnson, ed 3. p 137.)* Three quarters of patients with brain abscess have headache. This usually develops within a few weeks of the appearance of the abscess. Only a third of patients present with seizures or focal neurologic deficits. Only one-fourth exhibit papilledema. Brain abscesses may produce remarkably few changes in the CSF until the abscess penetrates into the subarachnoid or intraventricular space. Abscesses that have not yet communicated with the CSF will usually produce only a moderate elevation in the CSF protein content. If the abscess is unsuspected and untreated, it will usually extend to the ventricles. With perforation into the ventricle, the abscess usually proves fatal. The treatment of choice for brain abscess is surgical resection.

183. The answer is B. *(Johnson, ed 3. p 137.)* MR scanning is sensitive to the changes in brain tissues very early in the evolution of the brain abscess. CT scanning with contrast enhancement may reveal the typical picture of a lesion that is demonstrated as a ring, but the abscess may be quite advanced before this picture emerges. Substantial abnormalities of CSF composition are unlikely until the abscess perforates the ventricular wall. When perforation occurs, the CSF will exhibit numerous WBCs, a very high protein content, and a relatively low glucose content.

184. The answer is D. *(Rowland, ed 8. p 871.)* Patients with brain abscesses may exhibit focal signs, seizures, delirium, or less specific neurologic findings. Patients with brain abscesses often have fever, but the CSF may not reflect the infectious basis of the fever until the abscess ruptures into the ventricles or subarachnoid space. Although *Aspergillus* is the most common cause of fungal abscesses, it is a relatively uncommon cause of fungal meningitis or meningoencephalitis. *Nocardia* is not classified as a fungus despite its resemblance to a fungus.

185. The answer is A. *(Rowland, ed 8. pp 152–161.)* Tabes dorsalis is caused by *Treponema pallidum,* the agent responsible for all types of neurosyphilis, but it is a disease entity distinct from general paresis, the form of neurosyphilis in which personality changes and dementia do occur. With tabes dorsalis the patient develops a leptomeningitis. The posterior columns of the spinal cord and the dorsal root ganglia are hit especially hard by degenerative changes associated with this form of neurosyphilis.

186. The answer is B. *(Rowland, ed 8. pp 155–156.)* A gumma is a largely or entirely avascular granuloma. It rarely develops intracranially, but when it does it may grow to several centimeters across. The lesion starts as an inflammatory process but becomes fibrosed as it evolves. The term *gumma* has traditionally been reserved for granuloma-like lesions caused by spirochetal infection.

187. The answer is D. *(Davis, pp 655–659.)* General paresis is a slowly evolving process that may require years to produce substantial disability. Both the meninges and the parenchyma of the brain are involved by this chronic infection. In general paresis or paretic neurosyphilis, the meninges are thickened and opaque. A granular ependymitis characteristically develops. Degenerative changes occur throughout the cerebral parenchyma. Penicillin is the treatment of choice for this disease. The damage done to the brain is not mediated by autoimmune or adverse drug reaction mechanisms. This infection produces widespread injury to the brain, rather than the restricted brainstem damage that typically occurs with infections that attack structures arising from the embryonic rhombencephalon. With a rhombencephalitis, the pons and medulla oblongata are the principal targets of disease.

188. The answer is E. *(Adams, ed 4. p 590.)* Mumps, measles, and varicella zoster infection appear to be acquired primarily by way of the respiratory tract. The poliovirus is an enterovirus, which means it enters primarily through the gastrointestinal tract. Rabies is transmitted by animal bites and reaches the CNS by migration in neuronal processes presumably as it is swept along by retrograde axoplasmic flow. This is believed to be an unusual method of viral spread to the CNS. Most viruses that do produce CNS disease are carried to the CNS in the bloodstream rather than along neuronal processes with infected axoplasm.

189. The answer is E. *(Johnson, ed 3. p 121.)* Rabies is usually spread through the saliva of an infected animal. Introduction of saliva into a bite wound allows the virus to inoculate muscles or subcutaneous tissues. After introduction of the virus, the incubation period until fulminant infection appears extends from a few days to over a year, but usually ranges from 30 to 90 days. Animals transmitting the virus include dogs, bats, skunks, foxes, and raccoons.

190. The answer is D. *(Johnson, ed 3. p 121.)* Dehydration as a complication of rabies is no longer likely because intravenous fluids can be given to completely replace what the hydrophobic patient cannot consume by mouth. Other complications of rabies include a Guillain-Barré type syndrome in 20 percent of patients. Early after exposure, the patient will often complain of pain or paresthesias at the site of the animal bite. With the classic form of the disease, the patient will also exhibit intermittent hyperactivity.

191. The answer is A. *(Johnson, ed 3. p 125.)* No antiviral therapy affects the course of rabies. Immunization against rabies after exposure has occurred does not substantially improve the outlook. The infected patient must receive intensive care with precautions taken to prevent spread of the virus through contact with body fluids, such as saliva. Transmission of the virus through casual contact does not seem to occur, but it may be transmitted through corneal transplantation when the donor has been infected. Zidovudine (azidothymidine [AZT]) is an antiretroviral drug useful in slowing the progression of HIV-1 infection. Ganciclovir has found increasing use in the management of cytomegalovirus (CMV) infection, especially when CMV involves the eye in a chorioretinitis. Amantadine was developed as an anti-influenzal agent, but it is used primarily to reduce the symptoms of Parkinson disease. The reason for its antiparkinsonian action is unknown.

192. The answer is C. *(Adams, ed 4. p 23.)* Repetitive, large, sharp waves at about 1 Hz frequency may appear over the entire head as the patient with Creutzfeldt-Jakob disease develops profound dementia. This repetitive activity may appear as the patient develops prominent myoclonic jerks, but the repetitive EEG discharges are not muscle artifacts. Similar patterns occur with other types of encephalitis, but the association of periodic sharp waves with grossly disorganized background activity should suggest Creutzfeldt-Jakob disease, a slow-viral infection for which there is no treatment. Three per second spike-and-wave activity develops on the EEG of patients with generalized absence (typical petit mal) seizures. Triphasic waves, especially if they are most prominent frontally, occur most often with hepatic coma. An isoelectric EEG pattern may occur with barbiturate coma, profound hypothermia, or other transient conditions, but it is most often an indication of electrocerebral silence associated with cerebrocortical death.

193. The answer is D. *(Lechtenberg, Synopsis, p 100.)* Sensation is largely intact with Guillain-Barré syndrome. Some individuals complain of discomfort or paresthesias in the feet, but one of the fundamental characteristics of this rapidly ascending paralysis is the relative sparing of sensation. The weakness that evolves over the course of 2 weeks is usually quite symmetric, with proximal and distal musculature in the limbs equally involved. Tendon reflexes are invariably hypoactive or absent. That the corticospinal tracts are not significantly involved is evident from the lack of limb spasticity and the absence of an extensor plantar reflex response.

194. The answer is A. *(Adams, ed 4. p 13.)* The CSF in the patient with Guillain-Barré syndrome typically reveals an elevated protein content, varying from just over 100 mg/dL to well over 1000 mg/dL. The fluid does not have the pleocytosis typical of other paralyzing conditions such as poliomyelitis, but the mononuclear white blood cell count may be slightly elevated above the 5 to 10 cells/mm³ usually considered within normal limits. The CSF picture is sufficiently distinctive that for many years this syndrome was referred to as cytoalbuminemic dissociation, a designation that stressed the characteristic discrepancy between the elevation in albumin or protein level and relatively unremarkable cytologic features of the CSF. The glucose content of the fluid will be largely normal, another indication that bacterial infection is not responsible for the progressive paralysis.

195. The answer is B. *(Lechtenberg, Synopsis, p 100.)* The eye muscles are rarely involved with the Guillain-Barré syndrome except in a condition usually referred to as the Miller-Fisher variant. Muscle activity independent of the skeletal musculature—such as that in the iris, bladder, gastrointestinal tract, and heart—may be well preserved despite paralysis of the limb muscles, facial musculature, diaphragm, and voluntary oropharyngeal muscles. Bladder and bowel function and control may be largely intact even when the patient has lost all ventilatory control. Autonomic disturbances may produce excessive sweating and a mild tachycardia, but patients usually do not develop a life-threatening dysautonomia. Before adequate ventilatory support, patients died from the diaphragmatic paralysis that often develops.

Neoplasms

DIRECTIONS: Each question below contains five suggested responses. Select the **one best** response to each question.

196. Most of the brain tumors in children are

(A) metastatic lesions from outside the CNS
(B) oligodendrogliomas
(C) glioblastomas multiforme
(D) meningiomas
(E) infratentorial

197. Paramagnetic agents, such as gadolinium (gadopentatate dimeglumine), help to identify neoplasms on MR scanning of the head by

(A) enhancing the process of proton relaxation
(B) weakening the blood-brain barrier
(C) enhancing the radiopacity of perfused tissues
(D) lessening the contrast between gray and white matter
(E) enhancing the density of neoplastic tissue

198. The most common sources of primary brain tumors are

(A) glial cells
(B) neurons
(C) meningeal cells
(D) lymphocytes
(E) endothelial cells

199. A CNS tumor is considered primary if it

(A) can be found nowhere outside the brain
(B) can be found nowhere outside the CNS
(C) originated in the CNS
(D) originated in the embryonic brain
(E) originated outside the brain but spread exclusively to the brain

200. The most common type of primary brain tumor is

(A) meningioma
(B) astrocytoma
(C) lymphosarcoma
(D) oligodendroglioma
(E) medulloblastoma

201. The benign tumor likely to occur at the incisura of the tentorium cerebelli, on the falx cerebri, or overlying the planum sphenoidale is the

(A) osteosarcoma
(B) chondroma
(C) choroid plexus papilloma
(D) oligodendroglioma
(E) meningioma

202. The brain tumor most likely to develop with von Hippel–Lindau syndrome is

(A) glioblastoma multiforme
(B) meningioma
(C) hemangioblastoma
(D) ependymoma
(E) pinealoma

203. The most common tumor arising in the brain of the person with tuberous sclerosis is

(A) meningioma
(B) ependymoma
(C) optic glioma
(D) medulloblastoma
(E) astrocytoma

204. The most common source of metastatic tumors to the brain is the

(A) breast
(B) lung
(C) kidney
(D) skin
(E) uterus

205. Metastatic lesions to the brain most often appear

(A) at the gray-white junction
(B) in the thalamus
(C) in the posterior fossa
(D) in the caudate
(E) in the sella turcica

206. The tumor type common in the brain of patients with AIDS but otherwise extremely rare is

(A) lymphocytic leukemia
(B) metastatic lymphoma
(C) primary lymphoma
(D) Kaposi sarcoma
(E) lymphosarcoma

207. All the following metastatic brain tumors are radiosensitive EXCEPT

(A) lymphoma
(B) seminoma
(C) malignant melanoma
(D) breast carcinoma
(E) choriocarcinoma

208. The most common complication of a colloid cyst of the third ventricle is

(A) bitemporal hemianopia
(B) hydrocephalus
(C) gait ataxia
(D) optic atrophy
(E) oscillopsia

209. The shortest life expectancy with metastatic disease to the brain will be found in the patient with metastatic

(A) malignant melanoma
(B) breast cancer
(C) lung cancer
(D) renal cancer
(E) prostate cancer

210. Precocious puberty is most likely to arise with a tumor originating in the

(A) cerebellar vermis
(B) pineal body
(C) falx cerebri
(D) anterior commissure
(E) subthalamic nucleus

211. Bitemporal hemianopia is most likely to arise with

(A) an optic glioma
(B) an occipital astrocytoma
(C) a brainstem glioma
(D) a pituitary adenoma
(E) a sphenoid wing meningioma

212. Pituitary insufficiency may develop with any of the following EXCEPT

(A) craniopharyngioma
(B) choroid plexus papilloma
(C) giant aneurysm
(D) metastatic carcinoma
(E) hypothalamic glioma

213. With a posterior fossa ependymoma, the patient is at risk of dying because of

(A) transforaminal herniation
(B) emboli from the tumor
(C) vascular occlusion by the tumor
(D) hemorrhagic necrosis of the tumor
(E) status epilepticus

Neoplasms

Answers

196. The answer is E. *(Gilman, Disorders, p 333.)* The posterior fossa is the usual location for brain tumors in children. Medulloblastomas, ependymomas, and cerebellar or brainstem gliomas account for most of the tumors that occur before puberty. Other common tumors developing intracranially in children include optic gliomas and metastatic leukemias.

197. The answer is A. *(Adams, ed 4. p 17.)* In MR scanning the patient is surrounded by a powerful magnetic field that aligns protons in the water molecules of the body. A radiofrequency (RF) pulse disturbs the axis of alignment. As the protons return or relax to their initial configurations, the RF energy is released. The MR machine monitors and interprets this released energy and constructs a picture of the proton content of the tissues studied.

198. The answer is A. *(Lechtenberg, Synopsis, p 137.)* About 2 to 5 percent of all tumors occurring in the general population are primary CNS tumors. In adults, the most common primary brain tumor is the astrocytoma. In children, brain tumors are more likely to arise in the posterior fossa. Even in childhood, glial cell tumors, such as the cerebellar astrocytoma and the optic glioma, are common.

199. The answer is C. *(Lechtenberg, Synopsis, p 137.)* *Primary* has several meanings when used in reference to CNS disease. Whereas *primary* denotes an origin in the CNS structures (such as the brain and spinal cord) for a tumor, it denotes a genetic or idiopathic basis for a seizure disorder. A secondary seizure is one that is symptomatic of another process. *Secondary* is not the alternative to *primary* for brain tumors. With CNS neoplasms, the alternative to *primary* is *metastatic.*

200. The answer is B. *(Lechtenberg, Synopsis, pp 138–139.)* The most common primary brain tumors are malignant astrocytomas. These are classified as grade 3 or 4. Grade 4 astrocytoma is more commonly called *glioblastoma multiforme.* It is malignant in the very conventional sense that it invades adjacent tissue and metastasizes. This type of glial tumor is usually seen in adults; men are more susceptible than women.

201. The answer is E. *(Lechtenberg, Synopsis, pp 139–140.)* The incisura is formed by the tentorium cerebelli, which is itself a meningeal structure. The falx cerebri, also a meningeal structure, may give rise to meningiomas adjacent to the skull or deep-seated in the interhemispheric fissure. Meningiomas of the planum sphenoidale may impinge upon the optic chiasm and the patient may present with visual complaints, such as a bitemporal hemianopia.

202. The answer is C. *(Lechtenberg, Synopsis, pp 137–138.)* With von Hippel–Lindau syndrome the patient may exhibit tumors in multiple organs. In the brain, hemangioblastomas are the tumors most likely to arise, and these tumors are usually limited to the cerebellum or brainstem. Hemangioblastomas are often multiple and become symptomatic by bleeding into themselves. The initial episode of bleeding may prove lethal.

203. The answer is E. *(Johnson, ed 3. p 109.)* Giant cell astrocytomas develop in about 10 percent of patients with tuberous sclerosis. Other abnormal growths occur in the brain, and these are characterized as cortical tubers, neuronal heterotopias, and subependymal nodules. Rather than being neoplasms, these may be defects in cell migration or aggregation.

204. The answer is B. *(Lechtenberg, Synopsis, p 143.)* Breast, lung, kidney, skin, and uterus are all common sources of metastases to the brain. The incidences of metastases from the lung and breast in women are very close, but with climbing rates of pulmonary carcinoma in women, the lung has become the more common source. Skin lesions metastasizing to the brain include malignant melanomas.

205. The answer is A. *(Lechtenberg, Synopsis, p 143.)* Metastatic lesions are spread primarily by the vascular system. The gray-white junction is where the white matter and the gray matter meet. It is the interface at which blood-borne cells are most likely to lodge and grow. No part of the brain is exempt from the spread of metastases, but the cerebral hemispheres and the cerebellum are especially vulnerable.

206. The answer is C. *(Lechtenberg, AIDS, pp 99–109.)* Kaposi sarcoma is unusually common in patients with AIDS, but it is rarely metastatic to the brain. Metastatic lymphomas producing meningeal lymphomatosis are not especially rare in the general population, but primary lymphomas—that is lymphomas apparently arising in the CNS—were rare before the AIDS epidemic. The primary brain lymphoma usually presents as a solitary mass and can occur anywhere in the brain, but it does have a predilection for the periventricular structures.

207. The answer is C. *(Lechtenberg, Synopsis, pp 143–145.)* Lung cancers are variably responsive to radiation therapy, but protracted remissions can be achieved with some of these metastatic tumors to the brain with whole-brain irradiation. Irradiation is usually delivered over the course of several weeks with a total dose not usually exceeding 5000 rads to the whole brain. If the lesion may have spread beyond the brain, as is often the case with lymphocytic leukemia, irradiation of the entire craniospinal axis is appropriate.

208. The answer is B. *(Lechtenberg, Synopsis, p 142.)* Colloid cysts may produce transient or persistent obstruction of the flow of CSF. Because this is an especially deep-seated lesion, it may be more practical to simply shunt the fluid from the lateral ventricles rather than attempt to excise the cyst. These cysts are usually lined with epithelial cells and may arise from a variety of sources, including low-grade neoplasms that involute early in their evolution.

209. The answer is A. *(Lechtenberg, Synopsis, p 137.)* The outlook with malignant melanoma, breast cancer, lung cancer, or renal cancer metastatic to the brain is poor and limited to a matter of months, but malignant melanoma is especially grim because it is highly likely to bleed after it metastasizes to the brain. Malignant melanoma and choriocarcinoma are likely to produce lethal intracranial hemorrhages, and the former may in fact first become apparent only after it has precipitated an intracranial hemorrhage. Prostate cancer does not typically metastasize to the brain.

210. The answer is B. *(Lechtenberg, Synopsis, p 141.)* Tumors of several sorts arise in the region of the pineal. This is the usual site for the dysgerminoma or germinoma, a tumor of children not uncommonly associated with precocious puberty. This is a histologically benign tumor, but its location demands aggressive intervention to prevent the development of hydrocephalus and diencephalic dysfunction. Damage to the diencephalon in children will lead to a failure to thrive and ultimately death.

211. The answer is D. *(Lechtenberg, Synopsis, pp 141–142.)* With bitemporal hemianopia, the visual fields in both eyes are impaired, but only the temporal quadrants of the field in each eye are affected. Pressure on the optic chiasm inferiorly by a tumor arising in or near the sella turcica will crush the fibers crossing in the chiasm from the medial aspects of the optic nerves. The most medial fibers in both optic nerves are contributed by the nasal aspects of the retina. The nasal or medial aspects of the retina receive light from the temporal or lateral aspects of the visual field.

212. The answer is B. *(Lechtenberg, Synopsis, p 142.)* Choroid plexus papillomas usually develop intraventricularly and do not extend down into the sella turcica. These tumors affect both children and adults, but they are rare. They are benign if they are surgically accessible and are extirpated early in their evolution.

213. The answer is A. *(Lechtenberg, Synopsis, pp 140–143.)* As a posterior fossa tumor enlarges, the posterior fossa contents will be compressed and ultimately forced upward or downward. If the herniation is upward, it is called *transtentorial* because it is across the tentorium cerebelli. If it is downward, it is called *transforaminal* because it is across the foramen magnum. Ependymomas are not especially vulnerable to hemorrhagic necrosis. Tumors in the posterior fossa generally do not produce seizures.

Nutritional and Metabolic Disorders

DIRECTIONS: Each question below contains five suggested responses. Select the **one best** response to each question.

214. The enzymatic defect in Gaucher disease appears to be

(A) hexosaminidase B
(B) glucocerebrosidase
(C) phosphofructokinase
(D) glucose phosphorylase
(E) sphingomyelinase

215. All the following are considered sphingolipidoses EXCEPT

(A) Canavan disease
(B) Gaucher disease
(C) Niemann-Pick disease
(D) Krabbe disease
(E) Fabry disease

216. Encephalopathy develops with portal hypertension and chronic liver disease in adults because

(A) bilirubin levels in the blood produce kernicterus
(B) portal hypertension shunts toxin-laden blood into collaterals
(C) liver enzyme levels in the blood reach toxic levels
(D) concurrent anemia develops with the associated splenomegaly
(E) vitamin B_{12} cannot be processed in the damaged liver

217. The histologic feature in the brain most often seen with hepatic (portal-systemic) encephalopathy is

(A) an increase in Alzheimer type II astrocytes
(B) a loss of neurons
(C) microglial nodules
(D) neurofibrillary tangles
(E) plaque formation

218. The management of hepatic encephalopathy usually involves

(A) diphenhydramine
(B) ammonium chloride
(C) atropine
(D) dopamine
(E) neomycin

219. All the following are likely with uremic encephalopathy EXCEPT

(A) clouding of consciousness
(B) festinating gait
(C) asterixis
(D) dysarthria
(E) multifocal myoclonus

220. The CSF protein content with either uremic encephalopathy or hypertensive encephalopathy is likely to be

(A) abnormally low
(B) normal
(C) elevated to less than 100 mg/dL
(D) elevated to between 500 and 1000 mg/dL
(E) greater than 2000 mg/dL

221. The most common neurologic complication of chronic renal failure is

(A) peripheral neuropathy
(B) delirium
(C) seizures
(D) dementia
(E) labile affect

222. The restless legs syndrome that develops with uremia may be controlled with

(A) neomycin
(B) clonazepam
(C) amphotericin
(D) isoniazid
(E) rifampin

223. The most reliable treatment for the peripheral neuropathy of chronic renal failure is

(A) thiamine supplements
(B) clonazepam
(C) phenytoin
(D) minoxidil
(E) renal transplant

224. All the following occur with the dialysis disequilibrium syndrome EXCEPT

(A) mononeuropathy
(B) headache
(C) nausea
(D) muscle cramps
(E) obtundation

225. After renal transplantation, patients are at increased risk of developing

(A) glioblastoma multiforme
(B) meningioma
(C) primary brain lymphoma
(D) oligodendroglioma
(E) hemangioblastoma

226. For vitamin B_{12} to be absorbed, it must bind to

(A) a cyanide atom and form cyanocobalamin
(B) intrinsic factor
(C) the parietal cells of the stomach
(D) the ileal mucosa
(E) the jejunal mucosa

227. Deficiencies of vitamin B_{12} have their most obvious effects on the

(A) gastrointestinal system and the nervous system
(B) epithelial surfaces and the genitourinary system
(C) nervous system and the genitourinary system
(D) musculoskeletal system and the hematopoietic system
(E) hematopoietic system and the nervous system

228. The principal sites of neurologic damage with combined systems disease are

(A) the posterior and lateral columns of the spinal cord
(B) the anterior horn cells and spinothalamic tracts
(C) the nuclei gracilis and cuneatus
(D) the spinocerebellar and spinothalamic tracts
(E) Lissauer's tract and Clarke's column

229. All the following may be consequences of vitamin B_{12} deficiency EXCEPT

(A) myelopathy
(B) myopathy
(C) encephalopathy
(D) peripheral neuropathy
(E) optic atrophy

230. All the following may produce clinical syndromes similar to combined systems disease EXCEPT

(A) Lyme disease
(B) HIV-1
(C) HTLV-I
(D) herpes simplex
(E) nitrous oxide

231. The type of visual field cut most often seen with vitamin B_{12} deficiency is a

(A) centrocecal scotoma
(B) homonymous hemianopia
(C) bitemporal hemianopia
(D) binasal hemianopia
(E) hemianopia with central sparing

232. Persons with combined systems disease may have either hyporeflexia or hyperreflexia because

(A) different levels of the spinal cord are injured
(B) both anterior horn cells and corticospinal tracts are damaged
(C) both corticospinal and spinothalamic tracts are damaged
(D) both corticospinal tracts and peripheral nerves are damaged
(E) both cerebral and spinal neurons are damaged

233. With vitamin B_{12} deficiency there will be excessive urinary excretion of

(A) propionic acid
(B) succinic acid
(C) methylmalonic acid
(D) homocysteine
(E) pyruvate

234. Characteristics of Wernicke's encephalopathy include

(A) peripheral neuropathy
(B) receptive aphasia
(C) hyperreflexia
(D) anosmia
(E) ophthalmoplegia

235. Severe hypothyroidism may produce impaired consciousness with changes on the EEG consisting primarily of

(A) generalized slowing of background rhythm but with waves of normal configuration
(B) triphasic waves predominantly over the frontal areas
(C) spindles and K complexes
(D) spike-and-wave discharges with loss of all normal background activity
(E) recurrent burst suppression

Questions 236–238

A 37-year-old woman developed cholecystitis and required cholecystectomy. Her family advised the physicians involved that she had a long history of alcoholism and benzodiazepine use. Her drug use included diazepam (Valium), lorazepam (Ativan), and clonazepam (Klonopin). Approximately 7 days after the surgery, she became increasingly agitated, delusional, and suspicious. Routine investigations revealed no evidence of focal or systemic infection. Hepatic, renal, and hematologic parameters were largely normal. Within 24 h of her cognitive and affective changes she had a generalized tonic-clonic seizure. MR and CT studies of the brain were normal. Her CSF was unremarkable.

Answer the following questions with this clinical scenario in mind.

236. Her neurologic deterioration was most probably caused by

(A) a delayed anesthetic reaction
(B) benzodiazepine withdrawal
(C) alcohol withdrawal
(D) unreported cocaine use
(E) idiopathic epilepsy

237. In consideration of the abuse history provided by the family, medication orders prior to the surgery should have included

(A) haloperidol 1 mg PO for 3 days
(B) chlorpromazine 25 mg IM for 2 days
(C) trihexyphenidyl 2.5 mg PO for 3 days
(D) prochlorperazine 10 mg IM for 2 days
(E) thiamine 50 mg IM for 3 days

238. In anticipation of the seizures and cognitive deterioration that might occur postoperatively, the physician involved would have been wise to

(A) consult a psychiatrist and neurologist prior to surgery
(B) provide intravenous alcohol supplements postoperatively to blunt the alcohol withdrawal
(C) provide intramuscular or oral chlordiazepoxide several times daily at a dose dictated by the patient's level of agitation
(D) start phenytoin as a single dose nightly
(E) delay surgery until the risk of neurologic problems had abated

239. Syncope is likely with dysautonomia of the sort occurring in

(A) diabetes mellitus
(B) epilepsy
(C) multiple sclerosis
(D) Hallervorden-Spatz disease
(E) hypothyroidism

240. Premonitory signs of syncope include all the following EXCEPT

(A) shortness of breath
(B) tinnitus
(C) perioral paresthesias
(D) graying of vision
(E) déjà vu

241. A respiratory alkalosis is most likely involved in the syncope associated with

(A) uremia
(B) hyponatremia
(C) atelectasis
(D) pulmonary emboli
(E) hyperventilation

DIRECTIONS: Each group of questions below consists of lettered headings followed by a set of numbered items. For each numbered item select the **one** lettered heading with which it is **most** closely associated. Each lettered heading may be used **once, more than once, or not at all.**

Questions 242–248

For each of the following clinical scenarios, select the nutritional deficiency that is most likely responsible.

(A) Deficiency amblyopia
(B) Vitamin B_{12} deficiency
(C) Pyridoxine (vitamin B_6) deficiency
(D) Vitamin E (alpha-tocopherol) deficiency
(E) Vitamin D deficiency
(F) Thiamine (vitamin B_1) deficiency
(G) Nicotinic acid deficiency
(H) Kwashiorkor
(I) Vitamin C deficiency

242. A 26-year-old man developed hemoptysis and dyspnea over the course of 3 months. His physician suspected tuberculosis and started him on triple therapy with isoniazid (isonicotinic acid hydrazide), rifampin, and ethambutol. After 1 month of treatment, the patient's liver enzymes showed slight elevations, but the treatment was continued. The hemoptysis stopped by 2 months, but the patient complained of pins-and-needles sensations in his feet. Neurologic examination revealed hypoactive deep tendon reflexes in the legs and slightly impaired position sense. Strength was good in all limbs

243. A 50-year-old woman was found wandering in the street and was brought to the emergency room by the police. She was disoriented to time, place, and person, but had no evidence of head trauma. She staggered when she tried to walk, but she had no detectable alcohol in her blood. Eye movements were abnormal with paresis of conjugate gaze, and horizontal nystagmus was apparent. Relatives were contacted and they reported that this woman had a long history of alcohol abuse

244. A 46-year-old man complained of progressive visual problems. He noticed problems with discriminating objects both close and far away. His deficits progressed over the course of 3 months. He had a 12-year history of pipe smoking, a 14-year history of daily aspirin use, and a 20-year history of alcohol intake. He usually drank 4 ounces of gin daily. His examination revealed

enlargement of the physiologic blind spot to the point where it extended to central vision

245. A 32-year-old South African woman developed irritability, sleeplessness, and fatigue. Her family believed that she was depressed, but neurologic assessment established prominent short- and long-term memory problems. She had anemia and an obvious dermatitis on her face. Her diet was strictly vegetarian and limited almost entirely to grains, such as corn

246. A 61-year-old man developed progressive cramping of his legs and pins-and-needles in his feet over the course of a year. He consulted a physician when he noticed the paresthesias in his hands and unsteadiness of his gait. His family reported that he had had some urinary incontinence, but was too embarrassed to report it. On examination, he had a spastic paraparesis with severe disturbance of position and vibration sense in his legs. Despite obvious spasticity in the legs, the deep tendon reflexes were absent at the knees and ankles. His peripheral blood smear revealed hypersegmented polymorphonuclear leukocytes

247. A 4-year-old boy developed progressive gait ataxia and limb weakness over the course of 3 months. Neurologic assessment revealed diffusely absent deep tendon reflexes, proximal muscle weakness, ophthalmoparesis, and poor pain perception in his feet. Blood tests revealed elevated creatine kinase levels and abnormally high serum bilirubin levels. Further investigations of hepatic function revealed that the child had a cholestatic hepatobiliary disorder, but there was no evidence of hepatic dysfunction sufficient to cause an encephalopathy

248. A 9-month-old girl from famine-stricken Ethiopia exhibited profound apathy and indifference to her environment. She was afebrile and appeared to have no significant infections at the time of her initial evaluation. Her hair was sparse and slight edema was evident about her ankles. She was well below the 5th percentile for height in her age group. With handling she became irritable, but throughout her examination she exhibited little spontaneous movement. Her mother reported having seen transient tremors in the hands a few weeks earlier, but these had abated after a few days

Questions 249–254

For each of the clinical scenarios below, select the most likely diagnosis from the following list.

(A) Postictal state
(B) Hypothyroidism
(C) Uremic encephalopathy
(D) Wernicke's encephalopathy
(E) Herpes encephalitis
(F) Progressive multifocal leukoencephalopathy
(G) Meningeal carcinomatosis
(H) CNS toxoplasmosis

(I) Multiple sclerosis
(J) Hepatic encephalopathy
(K) Subacute combined systems disease
(L) Meningococcal meningitis
(M) Subacute sclerosing panencephalitis
(N) AIDS encephalopathy

249. A 23-year-old woman with a history of hemophilia noticed progressive memory difficulty. She had required little hematologic support, but she did require transfusion of factor VIII at least five times over the past 7 years. Neurologic examination revealed word-finding difficulty, poor recent and remote memory, gait ataxia, mild dysarthria, and a labile affect. Her right plantar response was extensor and her left brachioradialis reflex was hyperactive with transient clonus. An MR scan of the brain was unrevealing

250. A 19-year-old man developed obvious personality changes over the course of 2 weeks. He became agitated with little provocation and abused his wife both verbally and physically. His behavior was sufficiently atypical for him to prompt his relatives to seek psychiatric assistance for him. While being interviewed by a psychiatrist, he became unresponsive and developed generalized convulsions with opisthotonic posturing, tonic-clonic limb movements, and urinary incontinence. He was hospitalized for investigation of his seizure disorder. On initial examination he was noted to have a low-grade fever and a mild left hemiparesis. His CSF opening pressure was 210 mmH$_2$O. CSF cultures yielded no growth. His EEG revealed polyspike-and-wave discharges originating in the right temporal lobe. A CT of his brain revealed focal swelling of the right temporal lobe

251. A previously healthy 25-year-old woman developed acute loss of vision in her left eye. She awoke with pain in the eye and reduction of her acuity to perception of light and dark. She delayed seeing a physician for a week, during which time her acuity gradually improved sufficiently to allow her to read. On examination, the physician discovered she had slurred speech and poor rapid alternating movements with the left hand. Ocular dysmetria was evident in both eyes. Her tandem gait was grossly impaired. The physician obtained an EEG, which was normal

252. A 17-year-old man complained of headache and photophobia on awakening. His physician discovered a low-grade fever and resistance to neck flexion. He advised the patient to take acetaminophen and remain in bed for the next 24 h. Within 12 h the patient developed nausea and more intense headache. He seemed disoriented and inappropriately lethargic. His family brought him to an emergency room. The emergency room physician noted a petechial rash on the legs and marked neck stiffness. A CSF examination revealed a glucose content of 5 mg/dL, protein content of 87 mg/dL, and a cell count of 112 leukocytes, with 70 percent polymorphonuclear cells

253. A 56-year-old man was struck over the parietal area of the head during a robbery. He lost consciousness for 35 min but had no focal weakness or numbness on recovering consciousness. Within 2 days of the incident, his wife found him unresponsive in bed early in the morning. She called for an ambulance, but before it arrived her husband became more alert and asked for something to eat. He said he wanted to have some supper before he went to bed for the night. The ambulance attendant first on the scene noted that the patient was disoriented to place and time and had weakness of his right arm and leg

254. A 35-year-old woman was found unconscious on the floor of her apartment. A bottle of cleaning fluid was found on a table near her. One of the contents indicated in the fluid was carbon tetrachloride. The ambulance crew noted that the patient was breathing independently, but her breath had a distinctly fetid odor unlike that associated with the cleaning fluid. Her limbs were flaccid, and she groaned when she was moved. She responded to no inquiries and was poorly responsive to pain. A serum ammonia level obtained at the emergency room was 250 μg/dL, triple the normal level. An EEG revealed triphasic waves most prominently over the front of the head

Nutritional and Metabolic Disorders

Answers

214. The answer is B. *(Davis, pp 289–290.)* Gaucher disease produces hepatosplenomegaly and may cause lethal CNS disease. It is inherited as an autosomal recessive trait and may be diagnosed by demonstrating deficient glucocerebrosidase in fibroblasts or leukocytes. The severity of disease varies from nonneuronopathic types to acute infantile neuronopathic disease.

215. The answer is A. *(Davis, pp 286–287.)* The metabolic problem underlying Canavan disease is still unknown. It is not a sphingolipidosis because it does not involve a disturbance of sphingolipid metabolism or storage. All the sphingolipids are nothing more than lipids containing a sphingosine moiety. Sphingosine is a class of long-chain compounds with hydroxyl groups on carbons 1 and 3 and an amino group on carbon 2. They form ceramides by joining with fatty acids across the subterminal amino group.

216. The answer is B. *(Rowland, ed 8. p 861.)* Encephalopathy developing with chronic hepatic disease and portal hypertension is often called *portal-systemic encephalopathy* because of the importance of toxin-laden blood's bypassing the liver as portal hypertension develops. Precisely what toxins produce the encephalopathy is still debatable, but ammonia is probably one of the important ones, if not in fact the most important one. This type of encephalopathy will develop if flow through the liver is obstructed and the liver is otherwise normal. This is distinct from the terminal coma that may develop with acute hepatic necrosis.

217. The answer is A. *(Rowland, ed 8. p 861.)* Changes in the brain are notably sparse with portal-systemic encephalopathy. The Alzheimer type II astrocytes that increase in number are large cells. Rare patients show more dramatic changes, which do include neuronal loss and focal necrosis.

218. The answer is E. *(Rowland, ed 8. pp 862–863.)* Antibiotics are used with hepatic encephalopathy to reduce the number of intestinal bacteria that produce ammonia and other substances that are finally absorbed in the gut and act as neurotoxins. Lactulose is usually given in combination with neomycin at least in part to reduce the intestinal transit time of sources of nitrogen. In some institutions, metronidazole is given in addition to or instead of neomycin.

219. The answer is B. *(Rowland, ed 8. pp 867–868.)* A festinating gait is typically seen in patients with parkinsonism, and, although uremia can produce an enormous variety of neurologic signs, it does not typically produce a parkinsonian picture. Asterixis is an instability of hand and finger posture seen in both uremic and hepatic encephalopathy. This is also known as a "liver flap" because the patient has difficulty maintaining the hands in extreme extension and intermittently flexes them slightly, but abruptly, at the wrist.

220. The answer is C. *(Rowland, ed 8. p 868.)* In 60 percent of patients with uremic encephalopathy, the CSF protein content is greater than 60 mg/dL, but it exceeds 100 mg/dL in only 20 percent. The elevation with hypertensive encephalopathy is much more variable because intracranial hemorrhage may occur with the hypertensive crisis, but most patients will have protein changes of the magnitude seen with uremic encephalopathy. The increased protein level appears to develop with uremic encephalopathy because of greater permeability to proteins of the brain's capillaries when the patient is uremic. Dialysis may transiently correct the abnormality.

221. The answer is A. *(Rowland, ed 8. p 869.)* The type of peripheral neuropathy most commonly developing with chronic renal failure is a symmetric, distal, mixed sensorimotor neuropathy. The legs are generally affected first and most severely. Men are more commonly affected than women. Most of the peripheral neuropathies in patients with chronic renal failure involve axonal degeneration. The neuropathy usually improves with dialysis.

222. The answer is B. *(Rowland, ed 8. p 869.)* The restless legs syndrome is probably a harbinger of peripheral neuropathy. It is seen in patients with diabetes mellitus, as well as in those with chronic renal disease. The patient usually develops discomfort in the legs when trying to sleep. The dysesthesias associated with this syndrome include cramping and pruritus. Exercise before going to bed may alleviate much of the discomfort.

223. The answer is E. *(Rowland, ed 8. p 869.)* B vitamins are generally replaced when patients receive dialysis. Thiamine is water-soluble and so is easily lost during dialysis, but even replacing thiamine is not nearly as effective in retarding or reversing the neuropathy of chronic renal failure as is renal transplantation. There are presumed to be neurotoxins in the blood of patients with uremia that are not removed by routine dialysis.

224. The answer is A. *(Rowland, ed 8. pp 869–870.)* The sequelae of dialysis are generally signs of cerebral dysfunction. Occasionally these include convulsions and delirium. At its worst, dialysis disequilibrium may produce increased intracranial pressure with papilledema. This syndrome is presumed to develop as water shifts into the brain and out of the dialyzed blood.

225. The answer is C. *(Rowland, ed 8. pp 870–871.)* The primary brain lymphomas developing after renal transplantation may develop as late as 4 years after transplantation or as early as 5 months after transplantation. Primary brain lymphomas are usually sensitive to whole-brain irradiation, and patient survival for 3 to 5 years after the appearance of the tumor is fairly common. The tumor must be distinguished from the fungal and bacterial abscesses to which these transplant recipients are also susceptible. This susceptibility to opportunistic infections and brain lymphomas develops as a consequence of immunosuppressive therapy.

226. The answer is B. *(Davis, pp 396–397.)* Intrinsic factor is a glycoprotein secreted by the gastric parietal cells. In most people with vitamin B_{12} deficiency the problem is inadequate production of intrinsic factor, rather than inadequate vitamin B_{12} in the diet. Persons with pernicious anemia usually have an atrophic gastritis with inadequate intrinsic factor production as a consequence. This is presumed to be mediated by an autoimmune disorder.

227. The answer is E. *(Davis, p 398.)* The disease of the hematopoietic system associated with vitamin B_{12} deficiency is called *pernicious anemia* and that of the nervous system is *combined systems disease*. This vitamin is an essential cofactor in the conversion of L-methylmalonyl-CoA to succinyl-CoA and of homocysteine to methionine. Precisely how a deficiency of this vitamin causes combined systems disease, a disease affecting the spinal cord, is still unknown.

228. The answer is A. *(Davis, pp 398–399.)* The microscopic changes in the posterior and lateral columns of the spinal cord in the patient with combined systems disease include demyelination, gliosis, and vacuolar degeneration. The regions of the spinal cord most severely damaged are the lower cervical and upper thoracic. The vacuolar changes observed arise in the myelin sheaths of very large nerve fibers. Although this starts as a predominantly demyelinating lesion, it evolves into axonal loss.

229. The answer is B. *(Johnson, ed 3. p 365.)* The most common initial neurologic complaint with vitamin B_{12} deficiency is paresthesias in the feet with sparing of the hands. Vibration and position sense are disproportionately disturbed in the feet. Problems occur outside the nervous system, as well as throughout the central and peripheral nervous system. The most obvious disorder is hematologic with the appearance of a megaloblastic anemia.

230. The answer is D. *(Johnson, ed 3. p 365.)* HIV-1 and HTLV-I are retroviruses that may produce a myelitis. With HTLV-I, spasticity in the legs is more likely to be prominent than sensory changes, but both systems are affected. Prolonged nitrous oxide exposure is required to cause the combined systems–like disorder associated with this anesthetic agent. Lyme disease is caused by a treponeme and produces a range of neurologic problems similar to that caused by syphilis. In fact syphilis, as the cause of tabes dorsalis, is another consideration in patients with the clinical picture of combined systems disease.

231. The answer is A. *(Johnson, ed 3. p 366.)* The blind spot that normally occurs in each eye enlarges and extends temporally to involve central vision in patients with chronic vitamin B_{12} deficiency. This is similar to the blind spot associated with alcohol and tobacco excess, a problem called *tobacco-alcohol amblyopia*. Tobacco-alcohol amblyopia also seems to develop because of a vitamin B deficiency, but the deficiency is presumed to be thiamine rather than cobalamin.

232. The answer is D. *(Johnson, ed 3. p 365.)* Peripheral neuropathy of the sort occurring with vitamin B_{12} deficiency would ordinarily produce hyporeflexia. The lateral column damage, which involves the corticospinal tracts, would ordinarily cause hyperreflexia. Because both peripheral nerves and corticospinal tracts are damaged with vitamin B_{12} deficiency, the effect on reflexes is difficult to predict and often changes over time. The patient will usually start with hyperreflexia and develop either clonus or hyporeflexia.

233. The answer is C. *(Johnson, ed 3. p 366.)* Without sufficient vitamin B_{12}, the conversion of propionic acid to succinic acid is blocked and the intermediate compound, methylmalonic acid, accumulates in the blood. It is readily excreted and may help in the diagnosis of cobalamin deficiency when it is found in excess in the urine. Serum homocysteine levels may also be elevated because the conversion of homocysteine to methionine is disrupted if vitamin B_{12} is not available to expedite the methylation required.

234. The answer is E. *(Lechtenberg, Synopsis, pp 154–155.)* Peripheral neuropathy commonly develops with thiamine deficiency, but it is not a component of the encephalopathy caused by thiamine deficiency. A receptive aphasia develops in most persons who have suffered damage to the posterior two-thirds of the superior temporal gyrus. Cortical injuries do occur in the cerebellum of the alcoholic, but generally not in focal areas of the cerebrum. Because receptive aphasias are also known as *Wernicke's aphasias*, there may be confusion about their lack of relationship to Wernicke's encephalopathy. Hyporeflexia may develop as part of the peripheral neuropathy seen in patients with thiamine deficiency.

235. The answer is A. *(Adams, ed 4. pp 25–26.)* With endocrine disorders producing altered consciousness, the EEG is usually abnormal, but the abnormality may be little more than slowing of the background rhythm. The normal EEG background activity is alpha at 8 to 12 Hz. Mild slowing may shift the background to a theta rhythm at 4 to 7 Hz.

236. The answer is B. *(Lechtenberg, Seizure, pp 183–184. Lechtenberg, Synopsis, pp 44–45.)* The delay between surgery and the cognitive deterioration in this benzodiazepine-abusing patient was extraordinarily long to be accounted for by an adverse reaction to the anesthetic agent or to alcohol withdrawal. Paranoid delusions and seizures occurring with alcohol withdrawal are most likely during the first 72 h of abstinence. Benzodiazepine withdrawal may produce problems similar to those experienced with alcohol withdrawal, but a delay of 7 to 10 days between abstinence and the appearance of fulminant withdrawal symptoms is not atypical. Idiopathic epilepsy is not a reasonable diagnosis for a woman this age. Nothing in the history suggested cocaine abuse, but it is worth screening patients admitted with alcohol and benzodiazepine abuse for cocaine and amphetamine levels, especially if illicit drug use could complicate the hospitalization.

237. The answer is E. *(Lechtenberg, Synopsis, p 154.)* This woman was at risk for Wernicke's encephalopathy. She should have received supplemental thiamine for at least 3 days, even though this would not have prevented the cognitive deterioration that she exhibited. There was no indication for using a neuroleptic—like haloperidol, chlorpromazine, or prochlorperazine—even though her alcohol and benzodiazepine use placed her at risk for developing a withdrawal psychosis. The anticholinergic trihexyphenidyl was not appropriate as either a neuroleptic or an antiepileptic.

238. The answer is C. *(Lechtenberg, Synopsis, p 46.)* Chlordiazepoxide at relatively high doses of 25 to 100 mg four to six times daily will usually block the more malignant features of both alcohol and benzodiazepine withdrawal. This drug is itself a benzodiazepine, but once the patient has passed through the withdrawal period for the drugs he or she has been illicitly taking, the chlordiazepoxide can be systematically and uneventfully reduced. There are no apparent advantages to using an antiepileptic like phenytoin.

239. The answer is A. *(Johnson, ed 3. pp 19–20.)* Hypotension produces the syncope developing with diabetes mellitus. This is called *secondary autonomic insufficiency* because the problem is a consequence of peripheral nerve damage caused by the endocrine disorder. Other common causes of secondary dysautonomias include amyloidosis, porphyria, and vitamin deficiencies.

240. The answer is E. *(Lechtenberg, Synopsis, p 34.)* Distinguishing between seizures and syncope is occasionally difficult. Reports of déjà vu or jamais vu sensations just prior to a fleeting loss of consciousness suggest a complex partial seizure rather than a syncopal episode. After syncope, the patient should not have the confusion or focal deficits that may occur during a postictal period.

241. The answer is E. *(Lechtenberg, Synopsis, pp 35–36.)* With hyperventilation, carbon dioxide is rapidly cleared from the blood. With the ensuing syncope, hyperventilation ends and blood gases return to normal levels as the patient retains carbon dioxide. Hyperventilation syncope may be aborted by having the patient breathe into a closed container, such as a paper bag, so that carbon dioxide is rebreathed rather than expelled from the blood stream.

242. The answer is C. *(Adams, ed 4. p 820.)* Any patient treated with isoniazid must receive supplemental pyridoxine. Isoniazid does not interfere with pyridoxine absorption, but it does interfere with its participation in metabolic pathways. Persistently low pyridoxine activity leads to the development of a peripheral neuropathy. This is most likely to be seen as an isolated deficiency in patients on antituberculous therapy.

243. The answer is F. *(Adams, ed 4. pp 820–827.)* An apparently acute deterioration in cognitive function in an alcoholic may be from any one of several causes. Bleeding from esophageal varices may have produced a profound anemia. Inapparent head trauma may have produced a subarachnoid hemorrhage or subdural hematomas. If the patient's problem is from a nutritional deficiency, it is most likely from thiamine deficiency associated with alcoholism. That she has no alcohol in her blood at the time of the deterioration is irrelevant. The triad of dementia, gait difficulty, and oculomotor paresis is characteristic of Wernicke's encephalopathy, the rapidly progressive and potentially lethal form of thiamine deficiency.

244. The answer is A. *(Adams, ed 4. pp 830–831.)* The vitamin deficiency specifically responsible for injury to the optic nerve in persons who chronically smoke tobacco and drink ethanol is still uncertain. It probably arises from combined deficits of vitamins B_1, B_{12}, and riboflavin. This condition is also known as *nutritional optic neuropathy* and as *tobacco-alcohol amblyopia.* There has been considerable speculation about its arising as a consequence of chronic cyanide poisoning from tobacco smoking combined with vitamin B_{12} deficiency associated with alcoholism, but this theory has little support.

245. The answer is G. *(Adams, ed 4. pp 830–833.)* Persons with limited diet devoid of animal fats and rich in corn are at risk for pellagra, a nutritional deficiency of nicotinic acid or its precursor, tryptophan. This disease typically affects the skin, digestive tract, central nervous system, and hematopoietic system. People with diets limited to maize or corn are especially vulnerable because of the low levels of tryptophan and niacin in this grain.

246. The answer is B. *(Adams, ed 4. pp 833–836.)* The slow evolution of gait difficulty, bladder dysfunction, paresthesias, hyporeflexia, impaired position and vibration sense, and anemia suggests combined systems disease, the neurologic equivalent of pernicious anemia. Persons with this disease may have a diet rich in vitamin B_{12}, but if they lack intrinsic factor in the stomach, they will develop the deficiency. Patients usually acquire a megaloblastic anemia associated with the spastic paraparesis. Finding hypersegmented polymorphonuclear cells on the peripheral blood smear helps establish the diagnosis.

247. The answer is D. *(Adams, ed 4. p 836.)* Vitamin E deficiency causing neurologic disease is rare, but when it does develop it is usually during early childhood. The most common syndrome involves spinocerebellar degeneration, polyneuropathy, and pigmentary retinopathy. Clarke's columns, the spinocerebellar tracts, the posterior columns, the nuclei of Goll and Burdach, and sensory roots are especially likely to exhibit degeneration in persons with vitamin E deficiency.

248. The answer is H. *(Adams, ed 4. pp 840–841.)* Protein deficiency states, such as those occurring with kwashiorkor, produce a wide range of neurologic signs and symptoms. Although the CNS is somewhat sheltered from the ravages of malnutrition, severe protein-calorie deficiencies during childhood development may leave the child neurologically impaired for life. Even when dietary supplements have been introduced to correct the chronic deficiency, the children are likely to exhibit little improvement in mobility or alertness for weeks or months.

249. The answer is N. *(Lechtenberg, AIDS, pp 38–48.)* This woman is at relatively high risk for AIDS encephalopathy because she has required transfusion of clotting factors that have until recently been available only from pooled samples of blood products. The neurologic deficits that she exhibits are not specific for HIV-1 associated subacute encephalomyelitis (AIDS encephalitis) and are quite compatible with multiple sclerosis (MS). That her MR scan does not reveal plaques of demyelination scattered throughout the brain makes the diagnosis of MS improbable. To establish the diagnosis of AIDS encephalopathy, HIV-1 antibodies should be sought and the helper/suppressor (CD4/CD8) T-lymphocyte ratio should be checked. Patients with symptomatic AIDS usually have a CD4/CD8 T-lymphocyte ratio of less than 0.5.

250. The answer is E. *(Lechtenberg, Synopsis, pp 60–61.)* With herpes encephalitis in the person who is not immunodeficient, the first clinical signs of disease are likely to be psychiatric. Depression, irritability, and labile affect are especially common. The organic basis for the encephalopathy usually becomes self-evident when the affected person has a seizure. Because the temporal lobe is especially involved by herpes encephalitis, the initial seizure is likely to be complex-partial, but the seizure often becomes more generalized. The EEG will usually reveal the focal character of the cerebral damage. Intracranial pressure is usually increased with a fulminant infection. Temporal lobe swelling may be severe enough to produce lethal herniation.

251. The answer is I. *(Lechtenberg, Multiple Sclerosis, pp 37–44.)* Optic neuritis is often the first complaint that motivates the patient with multiple sclerosis to consult a physician. Clumsiness, stumbling, and other symptoms of ataxia are usually dismissed as inconsequential by the patient. Even individuals with profoundly slow and slurred speech are often unaware of their dysarthria. When the patient finally does consult a physician, multiple neurologic abnormalities are usually evident. This patient would be expected to have a positive swinging flashlight test (Marcus-Gunn pupil) and evidence of widespread demyelination on MR scan of the head.

252. The answer is L. *(Adams, ed 4. pp 555–561.)* With acute bacterial meningitis, the clinical progression may be limited to days between the first symptoms and death. A petechial rash developing over the lower parts of the body in the setting of fever, headache, nuchal rigidity, photophobia, and stupor must be considered presumptive evidence of a meningococcal meningitis. Rapid diagnosis and treatment is essential if the patient is to survive. The spinal fluid typically reveals a low glucose content, high protein content, and a leukocytosis with a large number of polymorphonuclear cells. Treatment with intravenous penicillin G 12 to 15 million units daily (divided into four to six doses) early in the course of illness may decide whether or not the patient survives more than a few hours or days.

253. The answer is A. *(Lechtenberg, Seizure, pp 67–69.)* After significant head trauma, the victim is at considerable risk for a seizure. A patient's seizure threshold is lowest when he or she is asleep or sleep-deprived. If the post-traumatic seizure occurs during sleep, it may go unnoticed. The patient's improving cognition suggested a postictal state. His hemiparesis was probably a Todd's paralysis, but any patient with posttraumatic seizures and focal weakness must be investigated for an acute or chronic subdural hematoma.

254. The answer is J. *(Adams, ed 4. pp 853–856.)* Carbon tetrachloride is a potent hepatic toxin. This woman may have attempted suicide by drinking cleaning fluid. As hepatic damage progressed she developed fetor hepaticus, a distinctive smell to her breath that reflects a profound metabolic disturbance. The serum ammonia level rose as liver function declined. The triphasic waves typically seen in hepatic encephalopathy may occur with uremia and other causes of metabolic encephalopathy.

Degenerative Disorders

DIRECTIONS: Each question below contains five suggested responses. Select the **one best** response to each question.

255. The most common cause of dementia in the general population is

(A) epilepsy
(B) vascular disease
(C) Alzheimer disease
(D) Parkinson disease
(E) head trauma

256. Pseudodementia in the elderly is most commonly caused by

(A) depression
(B) drug intoxication
(C) viral infection
(D) cerebral ischemia
(E) hypoxia

257. In the diseases causing dementia, myoclonus is usually most evident in

(A) Alzheimer disease
(B) Creutzfeldt-Jakob disease
(C) Parkinson disease
(D) Huntington disease
(E) Pick disease

258. In the dementia associated with Alzheimer disease, the EEG will usually show

(A) spike-and-wave discharges
(B) periodic frontal lobe discharges
(C) focal slowing
(D) generalized background slowing
(E) an isoelectric record

259. Pathologic features of Alzheimer disease are often seen in persons with

(A) multi-infarct dementia
(B) AIDS encephalopathy
(C) Wernicke's encephalopathy
(D) Behçet's disease
(E) Down syndrome

260. Chorea gravidarum only occurs in

(A) newborns
(B) depressed men
(C) pregnant women
(D) pubescent girls
(E) pubescent boys

261. Any of the following may produce chorea EXCEPT

(A) hypoxic brain damage
(B) ischemic brain damage
(C) olivopontocerebellar atrophy
(D) systemic lupus erythematosus
(E) hypothyroidism

262. Amyotrophic lateral sclerosis characteristically produces electromyographic changes that include

(A) fibrillations
(B) slow nerve conduction velocities
(C) impaired somatosensory evoked potentials
(D) f waves
(E) h reflexes

263. With Friedreich disease, all the following signs usually appear EXCEPT

(A) hyporeflexia
(B) truncal ataxia
(C) limb ataxia
(D) impaired position sense
(E) dementia

264. A 20-year-old ataxic woman with a family history of Friedreich disease developed polyuria and excessive thirst over the course of a few weeks. She noticed that she fatigued easily and had intermittently blurred vision. The most likely explanation for her complaints is

(A) inappropriate antidiuretic hormone
(B) diabetes mellitus
(C) panhypopituitarism
(D) progressive adrenal insufficiency
(E) hypothyroidism

265. The most prominent areas of degeneration with Friedreich disease are in the

(A) cerebellar cortex
(B) inferior olivary nuclei
(C) anterior horns of the spinal cord
(D) spinocerebellar tracts
(E) spinothalamic tracts

266. The peripheral neuropathy typically seen with Friedreich disease develops in part because of degeneration in

(A) dorsal root ganglia
(B) spinocerebellar tracts
(C) anterior horn cells
(D) Clarke's column
(E) posterior columns

267. The most common presenting complaint with Friedreich disease is

(A) visual loss
(B) syncope
(C) gait difficulty
(D) vertigo
(E) speech difficulty

268. Both Refsum disease, a disturbance of phytanic acid metabolism, and Friedreich disease cause all the following EXCEPT

(A) peripheral neuropathy
(B) sensorineural hearing loss
(C) pes cavus
(D) scoliosis
(E) retinal degeneration

269. In patients with either Roussy-Lévy syndrome or Dejerine-Sottas syndrome, biopsy of a peripheral nerve will typically reveal

(A) hypertrophic neuropathy
(B) demyelination
(C) axonal degeneration
(D) perineural infiltrates
(E) neurofibrillary tangles

270. With most types of olivoponto-cerebellar atrophy (OPCA), the pattern of inheritance of the disorder is

(A) sporadic
(B) autosomal dominant
(C) autosomal recessive
(D) sex-linked recessive
(E) mitochondrial

271. Pathologic characteristics of Alzheimer disease include all the following EXCEPT

(A) Lewy bodies
(B) neurofibrillary tangles
(C) neuronal atrophy
(D) senile plaques
(E) amyloid collections

272. If a parent has the gene for Huntington disease,

(A) half the offspring are at risk only if the affected parent is male
(B) half the offspring are at risk only if the affected parent is female
(C) half the offspring are at risk if either parent is symptomatic for the disease before the age of 30
(D) half the offspring are at risk for the disease
(E) one out of four children is at risk for the disease

273. Offspring of a parent with Huntington disease who develop rigidity and bradykinesia in adolescence probably have

(A) early-onset Huntington disease
(B) Parkinson disease
(C) postencephalitic parkinsonism
(D) drug-induced parkinsonism
(E) Wilson disease

274. On CT scanning of the brain of the patient with Huntington disease, atrophy is usually most evident in the

(A) cerebellum
(B) subthalamic nuclei
(C) putamen
(D) caudate
(E) substantia nigra

275. Huntington disease usually becomes symptomatic

(A) before puberty
(B) at puberty
(C) during adolescence
(D) during the third decade of life
(E) during the fourth or fifth decade of life

276. All the following are typical of Huntington disease EXCEPT

(A) labile affect
(B) loss of memory
(C) intention tremor
(D) impaired ocular fixation
(E) writhing and jerking movements of the limbs

277. Parkinsonism develops transiently with a variety of medications and chemicals, but irreversible signs of parkinsonism have occurred in persons who have taken

(A) 1-methyl-4-phenyl-1,2,3,6-tetrahydropyridine (MPTP)
(B) thioridazine (Mellaril)
(C) lysergic acid diethylamide (LSD)
(D) haloperidol (Haldol)
(E) reserpine

278. Even though the physiologic deficiency in Parkinson disease is of dopamine, L-dopa rather than dopamine is given to patients because

(A) L-dopa induces less nausea and vomiting than dopamine
(B) dopamine is readily metabolized in the gastrointestinal tract to ineffective compounds
(C) L-dopa is more readily absorbed in the gastrointestinal tract than is dopamine
(D) dopamine cannot cross the blood-brain barrier and therefore has no therapeutic effect in the central nervous system
(E) L-dopa is more effective at dopamine receptors than is dopamine itself

279. The affected person may exhibit any of the following as an early manifestation of Parkinson disease EXCEPT

(A) dementia
(B) oscillopsia
(C) tremor
(D) bradykinesia
(E) rigidity

280. Parkinsonism associated with neuroleptic use may be minimized if the patient receives adjunctive therapy with

(A) trihexyphenidyl (Artane)
(B) haloperidol (Haldol)
(C) methamphetamine
(D) thioridazine (Mellaril)
(E) L-dopa

281. After several years of successful antiparkinsonian treatment, a patient abruptly developed acute episodes of profound bradykinesia and rigidity with remission of these signs occurring as abruptly as the onset. This patient probably suffers from

(A) acute dystonia
(B) absence attacks
(C) on-off phenomenon
(D) complex partial seizures
(E) drug toxicity

282. The movement disorders seen with Parkinson disease include all the following EXCEPT

(A) cogwheel rigidity
(B) hemiballismus
(C) retropulsion
(D) masked facies
(E) shuffling gait

283. Communication is disturbed in persons with Parkinson disease because

(A) a receptive aphasia is common
(B) an expressive aphasia is common
(C) decrementing speech is typical
(D) echolalia is common
(E) dyslexia usually develops

284. Neurons remaining in the substantia nigra of the patient with Parkinson disease may exhibit

(A) intranuclear inclusion bodies
(B) intranuclear and intracytoplasmic inclusion bodies
(C) intracytoplasmic inclusion bodies
(D) neurofibrillary tangles
(E) amyloid plaques

285. All the following are useful in the management of Parkinson disease EXCEPT

(A) L-dopa/carbidopa combination (Sinemet)
(B) chlorpromazine (Thorazine)
(C) amantadine HCl (Symmetrel)
(D) benztropine (Cogentin)
(E) bromocriptine (Parlodel)

286. Carbidopa is used in combination with L-dopa because it

(A) has anticholinergic activity
(B) has dopaminergic activity
(C) is an antihistaminic
(D) is an antiemetic
(E) is a dopa decarboxylase inhibitor

287. The virus most likely responsible for postencephalitic parkinsonism is

(A) measles
(B) influenza
(C) mumps
(D) rubella
(E) herpes simplex

288. Progressive supranuclear palsy usually develops in

(A) childhood
(B) adolescence
(C) the third decade
(D) the fourth decade
(E) the fifth decade

289. The neurons most specifically damaged in amyotrophic lateral sclerosis (ALS) are

(A) sensory
(B) autonomic
(C) sympathetic
(D) parasympathetic
(E) motor

Questions 290–291

A 52-year-old man reported progressive weakness of his arms and legs over the course of 8 months. Examination revealed atrophy of muscles in the hands and forearms. Fasciculations were apparent in the tongue and in interosseus muscles of the hands. Tendon reflexes were hyperactive in both the arms and the legs. Clonus was evident at the right ankle, and the plantar response on the right foot was extensor. He had no sensory complaints and no apparent sensory deficits. He also had normal cognition.

With this clinical scenario in mind answer the following questions.

290. This man probably has a

(A) peripheral neuropathy
(B) encephalopathy
(C) myopathy
(D) myelopathy
(E) motor neuronopathy

291. Electromyographic studies on this man would be expected to reveal

(A) fibrillations
(B) slow conduction times
(C) good recruitment
(D) polyphasic waves
(E) electrical silence

292. Tics, or habit spasms, most commonly involve

(A) hemiballismus
(B) tongue biting
(C) obscene remarks
(D) eye blinking
(E) involuntary falls

293. Tourette syndrome is a disorder in which persons have any of the following EXCEPT

(A) multiple motor and vocal tics
(B) paranoid delusions and hallucinations
(C) obscene and scatologic vocalizations
(D) onset of disease by 21 years of age
(E) persistence of disease for more than 1 year

294. With Shy-Drager syndrome, syncope often occurs because of

(A) cardiac arrhythmias
(B) vertebrobasilar insufficiency
(C) orthostatic hypotension
(D) basilar impression
(E) hyperventilation

295. The cause of primary orthostatic hypotension is

(A) anemia
(B) idiopathic
(C) cardiac insufficiency
(D) degenerative central nervous system disease
(E) endocrinologic

296. Olivopontocerebellar atrophy usually develops in persons at risk because of

(A) neurotoxin exposure
(B) hereditary factors
(C) postencephalitic demyelination
(D) hypervitaminosis
(E) nutritional deficiencies

DIRECTIONS: The group of questions below consists of lettered headings followed by a set of numbered items. For each numbered item select the **one** lettered heading with which it is **most** closely associated. Each lettered heading may be used **once, more than once, or not at all.**

Questions 297–300

For each of the following clinical scenarios, pick the most likely diagnosis.

(A) Hepatolenticular degeneration	(G) Postencephalitic parkinsonism
(B) Hyperparathyroidism	(H) Butyrophenone effect
(C) Parkinson disease	(I) Phenothiazine effect
(D) Akinetic mutism	(J) Vegetative state
(E) MPTP poisoning	(K) Hypermagnesemia
(F) Locked-in syndrome	(L) Rhombencephalitis

297. A 34-year-old man developed progressive depression and memory impairment over the course of 6 months. His initial neurologic evaluation revealed a metabolic acidosis associated with his dementia. His liver was firm and his spleen appeared to be slightly enlarged. He had tremor and rigidity in his arms and walked with relatively little swing in his arms. His blink was substantially reduced, which gave him the appearance of staring. MR scanning of the brain revealed some atrophy of the putamen and globus pallidus. His cerebrospinal fluid was normal. His EEG was unremarkable

298. A 19-year-old woman developed auditory hallucinations and persecutory delusions over the course of 3 days. She was hospitalized and started on haloperidol (Haldol) 2 mg three times daily. Within a week of treatment she developed stooped posture and a shuffling gait. Her head was slightly tremulous and her movements were generally slowed. Her medication was changed to thioridazine (Mellaril), and trihexyphenidyl (Artane) was added. Over the next 2 weeks, she became much more animated and reported no recurrence of her hallucinations

299. A 65-year-old man developed slurred speech, difficulty swallowing, and labored breathing over the course of 30 min. When he arrived at the emergency room, he required ventilatory assistance. His arms and legs were flaccid and he exhibited no voluntary movements in any of his limbs. He was able to blink his eyes when instructed to and appeared to have completely intact comprehension of spoken and written language. An MR scan revealed extensive infarction of the lower pons, apparently associated with basilar artery occlusion

300. A 72-year-old man required bypass surgery to alleviate myocardial ischemia. During surgery, he had a massive myocardial infarct and protracted asystole. Resuscitative measures succeeded in reestablishing a normal sinus rhythm, but postoperatively the patient remained unconscious after 48 h. Over the ensuing weeks, the patient's level of consciousness improved slightly. He appeared awake at times, but did not interact in meaningful ways with visitors. He breathed independently and even swallowed food when it was placed in his mouth, but he remained mute. With painful stimuli he exhibited semipurposeful withdrawal of his limbs. His clinical status remained unchanged for several more months

DIRECTIONS: The group of questions below consists of four lettered headings followed by a set of numbered items. For each numbered item select

A	if the item is associated with	(A) **only**
B	if the item is associated with	(B) **only**
C	if the item is associated with	**both** (A) and (B)
D	if the item is associated with	**neither** (A) nor (B)

Each lettered heading may be used **once, more than once, or not at all.**

Questions 301–304

(A) Alzheimer disease
(B) Pick disease
(C) Both
(D) Neither

301. Personality structure deteriorates rapidly and constructional difficulties develop early in the evolution of the dementia and are prominent features of the syndrome

302. Cortical atrophy is usually evident on CT or MR scanning

303. Seizures commonly occur with the cortical degeneration

304. Changes in the caudate nucleus may be similar to those found with Huntington disease

Degenerative Disorders
Answers

255. The answer is C. *(Lechtenberg, Synopsis, pp 65–66. Rowland, ed 8. pp 5–7.)* Alzheimer disease accounts for as much as 50 percent of the dementia in the general population confirmed at autopsy. Parkinson disease accounts for only about 1 percent. Only 80 years ago, neurosyphilis was the most common cause of dementia, but the introduction of penicillin reduced, though it did not eliminate, this spirochetal disease as a cause of dementia. As the population ages, the incidence and prevalence of Alzheimer disease are increasing. The dementia caused by Alzheimer disease is progressive over the course of years. Language disturbances may appear even before memory problems.

256. The answer is A. *(Rowland, ed 8. pp 7–8.)* Pseudodementia is cognitive impairment not caused by a structural, metabolic, infectious, or otherwise organic problem. Depression in the elderly may produce many of the signs and symptoms of a true dementia, but treating the depression alone will correct the dementia. This is not a contrived or fictitious dementia. The impairment in performance is involuntary and amenable to treatment with antidepressants.

257. The answer is B. *(Rowland, ed 8. p 8.)* Creutzfeldt-Jakob disease is a slow-viral illness that produces dementia over the course of months. Myoclonic jerks, abrupt involuntary muscle contractions that may produce brief limb or facial movements, usually appear at some time in the course of this disease. Similar movements may develop with Huntington disease, but these patients usually develop more constant and fluid limb movements called *chorea*.

258. The answer is D. *(Rowland, ed 8. p 8.)* The background rhythm on the normal adult EEG is alpha activity at 8 to 12 Hz. With Alzheimer disease the frequency of this rhythm may slow and the amount of time this rhythm is evident when the patient is lying relaxed with eyes closed may drop substantially. Periodic discharges in the form of sharp waves or spikes may develop during Creutzfeldt-Jakob disease. The EEG is otherwise not especially helpful in distinguishing between the common causes of dementia.

259. The answer is E. *(Lechtenberg, Synopsis, pp 65–66.)* The senile plaques, neurofibrillary tangles, and neuronal dropout characteristically seen with Alzheimer disease appear in most persons dying as adults with trisomy 21. The Down syndrome patients develop these pathologic features decades before they are usually obvious in the patient with Alzheimer disease. The relationship between the two diseases is not understood.

260. The answer is C. *(Lechtenberg, Synopsis, p 87.)* *Chorea gravidarum* designates an involuntary movement disorder occurring during pregnancy and involving relatively rapid and fluid, but not rhythmic, limb and trunk movements. This type of movement disorder may also appear with estrogen use, but the fundamental problem is a dramatic change in the hormonal environment of the brain. At the end of pregnancy or with the withdrawal of the offending estrogen, the movements abate. The movements developing with chorea gravidarum may be quite asymmetric and forceful.

261. The answer is E. *(Lechtenberg, Synopsis, pp 85–86.)* Although hyperthyroidism may produce involuntary movements reminiscent of chorea, hypothyroidism should not be adopted as an explanation for chorea if it appeared in a patient with this type of thyroid disorder. Causes of chorea include multiple sclerosis, hypoxic brain damage, ischemic brain damage, systemic lupus erythematosus, olivopontocerebellar atrophy, and encephalitis. Endocrine problems other than hyperthyroidism, such as hypoadrenalism, may also produce chorea.

262. The answer is A. *(Adams, ed 4. p 37. Lechtenberg, Synopsis, pp 25–26.)* Fibrillations are evidence of anterior horn cell disease. They are usually associated with fasciculations, but unlike fasciculations the muscle activity associated with fibrillations is not obvious on inspection of the muscle. A fibrillation is a low-amplitude, high-frequency muscle action potential unprovoked by voluntary activity. It is limited to a single muscle fiber and exerts too little force to produce any movement of the joint. Muscle atrophy usually accompanies fibrillations and fasciculations in the person with amyotrophic lateral sclerosis (ALS).

263. The answer is E. *(Rowland, ed 8. p 627.)* Friedreich disease, or ataxia, is a recessively transmitted degenerative disorder. It usually becomes symptomatic in the first or second decade of life. Patients often develop scoliosis and clubfoot as the disorder progresses.

264. The answer is B. *(Rowland, ed 8. p 627.)* More than 10 percent of patients with Friedreich disease develop diabetes mellitus. A more life-threatening complication of this degenerative disease is the disturbance of the cardiac conduction system that often develops. Visual problems occur with the hyperglycemia of uncontrolled diabetes mellitus, but even patients without diabetes develop optic atrophy late in the course of the degenerative disease.

265. The answer is D. *(Rowland, ed 8. p 627.)* Degeneration is primarily in the spinal cord rather than the cerebellum or brainstem in patients with Friedreich disease. Both the dorsal and ventral spinocerebellar tracts are involved. The other spinal cord structures exhibiting degeneration include the posterior columns and the lateral corticospinal tracts.

266. The answer is A. *(Rowland, ed 8. pp 627–628.)* Degenerative changes in the peripheral nerves of patients with Friedreich disease have several bases. Loss of cells in the dorsal root ganglia makes a major contribution to this phenomenon. Additional sites of degeneration affecting the sensory system include the substantia gelatinosa (Lissauer's tract) of the posterior horn and the dorsal roots themselves. The peripheral neuropathy is responsible for the hyporeflexia that is invariably found in the legs of affected persons.

267. The answer is C. *(Gilman, Disorders, p 239.)* Gait difficulty usually develops during childhood in persons with Friedreich disease. Visual loss, syncope, vertigo, and dysarthria may develop during the course of this degenerative disease, but the appearance of these other problems may be decades after that of the gait ataxia. Visual loss may develop with optic atrophy or retinitis pigmentosa.

268. The answer is B. *(Gilman, Disorders, p 241.)* Refsum disease is inherited in an autosomal recessive manner. Clumsiness and gait ataxia are the initial complaints of this disease, and most victims of the disease become symptomatic early in childhood. The hearing loss that develops with Refsum disease may be apparent very early in the course of the degeneration. Cardiac complications occur in both this type of degenerative disorder and Friedreich disease.

269. The answer is A. *(Gilman, Disorders, p 243.)* The myelin sheaths about the nerve fibers in Roussy-Lévy syndrome and Dejerine-Sottas syndrome, both idiopathic causes of peripheral neuropathy, have an excess number of layers. With Dejerine-Sottas the patient's complaints refer to this peripheral neuropathy almost exclusively. With Roussy-Lévy, the picture is complicated by severe ataxia, tremor, and pes cavus.

270. The answer is B. *(Gilman, Disorders, pp 244–246.)* Unlike Friedreich disease, the onset of OPCA may be fairly late in life. Most patients become symptomatic after the third decade of life. The cerebellum is very directly involved by atrophy in this dominantly inherited degenerative disorder. Dementia may be evident in some variants. Ocular problems, including ophthalmoplegia and optic atrophy, are also fairly common.

271. The answer is A. (*Lechtenberg, Synopsis, pp 65–66.*) Lewy bodies typically occur in cells of the substantia nigra in Parkinson disease. With Alzheimer disease, there are no characteristic inclusion bodies, but amyloid material does accumulate in the brain parenchyma in senile plaques. Neurofibrillary tangles, which develop in axons and dendrites, and neuronal loss, which may be widespread throughout the cerebral cortex, are found in patients with Alzheimer disease, but the cause is unknown.

272. The answer is D. (*Lechtenberg, Synopsis, pp 86–87.*) Huntington disease is transmitted in an autosomal dominant fashion. The age at which the patient becomes symptomatic is variable and has no effect on the probability of transmitting the disease. The defect underlying this degenerative disease is transmitted on chromosome 4.

273. The answer is A. (*Lechtenberg, Synopsis, p 87.*) The rigid form of Huntington disease is sometimes referred to as *Westphal disease* or *Westphal variant*. This form usually presents earlier in life than the chorea more typically seen with Huntington disease. Dementia and affective disorders develop with classic Huntington disease and this variant.

274. The answer is D. (*Lechtenberg, Synopsis, p 87.*) The head of the caudate is usually atrophic early in the course of Huntington disease. This is readily seen on CT scanning because the head of the caudate gives the lateral ventricle its typical comma or boomerang appearance. As the caudate atrophies, the frontal tip of the lateral ventricle becomes increasingly rhomboidal in shape.

275. The answer is E. (*Davis, p 792.*) Only 5 to 10 percent of patients with Huntington disease become symptomatic before the second decade of life. Sporadic cases may even appear during early childhood or during senescence. The earliest signs of disease may include either disturbed thinking or movements.

276. The answer is C. (*Davis, pp 792–793.*) Tremor on activity or intended activity is more typically seen in patients with progressive cerebellar disease than in those with Huntington disease. The person with Huntington disease has evidence of extensive basal ganglia disease. In fact, both the caudate and the putamen are severely atrophic. Cerebral cortical atrophy is routinely present, but it is generally most prominent in the frontal and temporal lobes.

277. The answer is A. *(Adams, ed 4. p 59.)* Efforts to make an opiate resulted in the toxin MPTP. Young adults who self-administered this drug developed progressive damage to the substantia nigra and exhibited the typical signs of rigidity, tremor, and bradykinesia seen with idiopathic Parkinson disease. That a toxin can produce a syndrome indistinguishable from Parkinson disease has increased speculation that some, and perhaps many, persons with Parkinson disease have had environmental exposure to a toxin that produced degeneration of the substantia nigra.

278. The answer is D. *(Adams, ed 4. p 59.)* L-Dopa crosses the blood-brain barrier easily and is subsequently converted to dopamine in the CNS. Conversion of L-dopa to dopamine occurs outside the CNS in a wide variety of tissues, but once converted to dopamine in the periphery the drug becomes inaccessible to the brain. Peripheral conversion of L-dopa to dopamine is routinely inhibited by adding a dopa-decarboxylase inhibitor to the therapeutic regimen. Carbidopa, the inhibitor most widely used, does not penetrate the blood-brain barrier substantially. Because it is largely excluded from the CNS, carbidopa cannot inhibit the conversion of L-dopa to dopamine in the brain.

279. The answer is B. *(Gilman, Disorders, p 193.)* Oscillopsia occurs with cerebellar damage and is not characteristic of any degenerative disease of basal ganglia. Patients with this complaint describe environmental oscillations that often coincide with obvious nystagmus. Similar complaints may develop in patients with damage to the labyrinth of the inner ear.

280. The answer is A. *(Lechtenberg, Synopsis, p 78.)* Trihexyphenidyl (Artane) is an anticholinergic drug. It is presumed to decrease signs of parkinsonism caused by drugs that interfere with dopamine neurotransmission by creating a relative deficiency of acetylcholine neurotransmission. In a very simplistic view of the CNS, the cholinergic and dopaminergic systems have antagonistic actions.

281. The answer is C. *(Lechtenberg, Synopsis, pp 76–79.)* The on-off effect is commonly seen in persons who have had Parkinson disease for several years. Maintaining more stable levels of antiparkinsonian medication in the blood does not eliminate this phenomenon of abruptly worsening and remitting symptoms. Variability in the responsiveness of the CNS to the medication, rather than variability in the medication levels, underlies the phenomenon.

282. The answer is B. *(Davis, p 799.)* Hemiballismus typically occurs with subthalamic damage. Movement problems in Parkinson disease other than those listed include pill-rolling tremor, stooped posture, and anteropulsion, an inability to stop walking once a regular pace has been achieved. Retropulsion is an exaggerated tendency to fall backward. Posture and postural stability are major problems for the person with Parkinson disease.

283. The answer is C. *(Davis, p 799.)* Speech volume tapers off as the person with parkinsonism speaks. Later in the disease speech may be reduced to a whisper at all times. Writing deteriorates in much the same way as speech. Micrographia routinely develops in patients with Parkinson disease.

284. The answer is C. *(Davis, p 799.)* The intracytoplasmic inclusion bodies commonly seen in patients with idiopathic Parkinson disease are called Lewy bodies. They are eosinophilic inclusions with poorly staining halos surrounding them. They may be round or oblong in shape and are most common in the substantia nigra, locus ceruleus, and substantia innominata. They appear to consist of aggregated neurofilaments. Degenerative changes may be remarkably asymmetric in patients with Parkinson disease.

285. The answer is B. *(Lechtenberg, Synopsis, pp 76–79.)* Chlorpromazine is a phenothiazine. Phenothiazines and butyrophenones, such as haloperidol (Haldol), worsen parkinsonism in patients with Parkinson disease and produce signs of parkinsonism in persons without Parkinson disease. Amantadine is an antiviral agent that helps reduce the signs of parkinsonism, but its mechanism of action is unclear. Bromocriptine has a dopaminergic effect on postsynaptic membranes.

286. The answer is E. *(Lechtenberg, Synopsis, pp 76–79.)* Dopa decarboxylase converts L-dopa to dopamine. Carbidopa crosses the blood-brain barrier poorly, and so its inhibition of this enzyme is restricted to activity outside the CNS. Conversion of L-dopa to dopamine continues to occur in the CNS when the patient takes Sinemet.

287. The answer is B. *(Lechtenberg, Synopsis, p 79.)* After the epidemic of encephalitis lethargica of 1918 to 1926, there were many cases of postencephalitic parkinsonism. The causative agent was believed to be an influenza virus, but the causative agent could not be isolated with the techniques available at the time of the epidemic. Postinfluenzal parkinsonism still develops, but the incidence is too rare to establish that this virus is the only virus capable of producing parkinsonism.

288. The answer is E. *(Davis, p 803.)* Men are affected much more often than women by progressive supranuclear palsy (PSP). The disease evolves over the course of years. The most common initial complaint is a problem with looking downward. Eventually the patient loses all vertical eye movements. Signs of parkinsonism accompany the ocular motor disturbance.

289. The answer is E. *(Lechtenberg, Synopsis, p 101.)* ALS is often called *motor neuron disease* precisely because it so dramatically targets the motor neurons. Damage to the motor system produces wasting, weakness, and spasticity. If cranial musculature is affected early in the course of the disease, the patient's survival is more likely to be curtailed.

290. The answer is E. *(Lechtenberg, Synopsis, p 101.)* Amyotrophic lateral sclerosis (ALS), a motor neuron disease, best explains this clinical scenario. Because bulbar involvement evolved during the first year of disease in the patient described, the prognosis is poor. Survival for more than a year or two from this point in the clinical evolution is unlikely. Death usually results from respiratory complications, such as aspiration pneumonia or ventilatory arrest.

291. The answer is A. *(Adams, ed 4. p 37.)* Fibrillations are action potentials of very small amplitude that appear with anterior horn cell disease. They occur independently of voluntary muscle contractions. With ALS, fibrillations will be apparent in muscles with no apparent atrophy, as well as in those with substantial atrophy. The electrical activity recorded is the isolated activity of individual muscle fibers, perhaps triggered by denervation hypersensitivity.

292. The answer is D. *(Lechtenberg, Synopsis, p 85.)* Common tics include shoulder shrugs, head tosses, and facial grimaces, as well as eye blinks. These are all, by definition, involuntary, repetitive movements that are usually quite brief. Concentration on the activity may suppress it temporarily, but the patient with a tic will feel increasing tension the longer he or she tries to suppress the involuntary movement.

293. The answer is B. *(Lechtenberg, Synopsis, p 85.)* With Tourette syndrome there appears to be an autosomal dominant pattern of inheritance with variable penetrance. Most of the affected persons are men. A variety of drugs may help suppress the tics that are characteristic of this syndrome. These include haloperidol, pimozide, trifluoperazine, and fluphenazine.

294. The answer is C. *(Lechtenberg, Synopsis, pp 34–35.)* Shy-Drager is a syndrome affecting men in their thirties, forties, and fifties in which progressive autonomic failure develops. The sympathetic nervous system deteriorates over the course of years. The most common initial complaint in affected persons is impotence. Problems with sweating and bowel motility are also usually early signs of this dysautonomia.

295. The answer is B. *(Lechtenberg, Synopsis, p 35.)* Orthostatic hypotension may develop with degenerative, nutritional, cardiac, or hematologic disease. If all these potential causes can be excluded, the disorder is defined as primary. The most common cause of orthostatic hypotension is actually iatrogenic. Overmedication with or excessive sensitivity to antihypertensive agents produces much of the orthostatic hypotension that warrants medical attention.

296. The answer is B. *(Gilman, Disorders, pp 244–250.)* Most olivopontocerebellar atrophies are transmitted in an autosomal dominant fashion. Many are linked to a defective gene on chromosome 6. These disorders are distinct from Friedreich disease. In the latter, neuropathologic changes are much less prominent in the cerebellum than they are with OPCA. The gene defect responsible for Friedreich disease has been traced to chromosome 9.

297. The answer is A. *(Lechtenberg, Synopsis, p 80.)* Hepatolenticular degeneration (Wilson's disease) often becomes symptomatic in the second or third decade of life, but its initial presentation may be delayed until the fourth or fifth decade. Renal tubular acidosis develops along with hepatic fibrosis. Systemic problems include heart and lung damage, but most patients become most symptomatic from their brain and liver disease. Dementia is progressive if the patient is not treated. Hepatic disease will progress to hepatic failure if the patient is left untreated. Appropriate treatment includes the chelating agent penicillamine, which depletes the body of copper.

298. The answer is H. *(Lechtenberg, Synopsis, pp 79–80.)* Butyrophenones, the most commonly prescribed of which is haloperidol, routinely produce some signs of parkinsonism if they are used at high doses for more than a few days. This psychotic young woman proved to be less sensitive to the parkinsonian effects of the phenothiazine thioridazine than she was to haloperidol. Adding the anticholinergic trihexyphenidyl may also have helped to reduce the patient's parkinsonism.

299. The answer is F. *(Lechtenberg, Synopsis, p 29.)* Consciousness is preserved in the locked-in syndrome, but the patient is paralyzed from the eyes down. Survival is usually limited to days or weeks in patients with this clinical syndrome. In most cases the locked-in syndrome develops because of ischemic or hemorrhagic damage to the pons, such as that occurring with basilar artery occlusion.

300. The answer is J. *(Lechtenberg, Synopsis, p 31.)* The vegetative state is a clinical condition in which autonomic activity is sustained with little evidence of cognitive function. With protracted asystole the patient may have extensive damage to the cerebral cortex with little damage to the brainstem. The ischemic damage to the cerebrum should be evident on MR scanning soon after the injury. This type of damage is usually responsible for the appearance of the vegetative state. It also may develop with drowning or other causes of protracted hypoxia.

301–304. The answers are: 301-B, 302-C, 303-D, 304-B. *(Davis, p 789.)* With Pick disease, patients have prominent signs of frontal and parietal lobe damage early in the course of disease. These patients have much less insight into their deterioration than do patients with slowly evolving Alzheimer disease, and consequently they exhibit considerably less depression early in the course of disease. Memory disturbances and mood fluctuations are common in patients with both Pick and Alzheimer disease.

With Pick disease the apparent atrophy is more localized than that seen on CT or MR scan in the patient with Alzheimer disease. The frontal lobe atrophy is especially evident. The posterior two-thirds of the superior temporal gyrus may be strikingly spared in Pick disease. The atrophy in both diseases results from several structural changes in the brain, which include neuronal loss. Some of the surviving neurons in Pick disease may have cytoplasmic inclusion bodies that stain with silver stains. These are called *Pick bodies.*

Although seizures are a common sign of cortical disease, neither Pick nor Alzheimer disease commonly elicits seizure activity in affected persons. Rigidity and abnormal movements are also relatively uncommon in both of these diseases. Survival with both conditions is measured in years, and survival past 5 years from onset of symptoms is not unusual. Death usually occurs because of inanition, dehydration, or chronic infection.

Although atrophy of the caudate may be extreme with Pick disease, the putamen is generally not as damaged. Other elements of the basal ganglia, including the globus pallidus and substantia nigra, are variably affected in Pick disease. Neuronal loss is most striking in the cortex with Pick disease; the outer three layers of the cortex are most notably involved.

Demyelinating Disorders

DIRECTIONS: Each question below contains five suggested responses. Select the **one best** response to each question.

305. Multiple sclerosis is the most common demyelinating disease in the United States and as such affects approximately 1 person in

(A) 100
(B) 500
(C) 1000
(D) 5000
(E) 10,000

306. Multiple sclerosis is usually diagnosed on the basis of several pieces of evidence that may include all the following EXCEPT

(A) recurrent episodes of tonic-clonic seizure activity
(B) elevated CSF gamma globulin content
(C) neuroimaging evidence of multifocal demyelination
(D) recurrent episodes of optic neuritis
(E) progressive bladder dysfunction

307. All the following are demyelinating disorders EXCEPT

(A) general paresis
(B) multiple sclerosis
(C) subacute sclerosing panencephalitis
(D) progressive multifocal leukoencephalopathy
(E) metachromatic leukodystrophy

308. A papovavirus infection of the CNS in an immunodeficient person is most likely to produce

(A) adrenoleukodystrophy
(B) multiple sclerosis
(C) subacute sclerosing panencephalitis
(D) progressive multifocal leukoencephalopathy
(E) metachromatic leukodystrophy

309. MR scanning reveals demyelinated plaques much more clearly than CT scanning because

(A) myelin has a greater density than gray matter
(B) the water content but not the density of tissue changes substantially with demyelination
(C) there is relative ischemia in regions of extensive demyelination
(D) MR is more sensitive to changes in white matter than gray matter
(E) the ionizing radiation used for CT scanning produces confounding artifacts in white matter

310. The CSF in persons with multiple sclerosis will typically exhibit

(A) glucose content of less than 20 percent of the serum content
(B) persistently elevated total protein content
(C) persistently elevated immunoglobulin G (IgG) content
(D) mononuclear cell counts of greater than 100 cells per cubic millimeter
(E) erythrocyte counts of greater than 10 cells per cubic millimeter

311. Oligoclonal bands are the

(A) wave frequency changes on the EEG during sleep
(B) markings about the iris seen in Wilson disease
(C) pathologic features of Alzheimer disease
(D) chromosomal markings found with MS
(E) immunoglobulin patterns in the CSF with MS

312. The diagnostic method LEAST likely to provide evidence to support the diagnosis of MS is

(A) visual evoked responses
(B) serum protein electrophoresis
(C) CT scanning of the brain with double-dose contrast enhancement
(D) MR scanning of the brain
(E) somatosensory evoked potentials

313. In comparison with acute exacerbations of MS left untreated, those treated with adrenocorticotropic hormone (ACTH)

(A) result in less permanent disability
(B) do not produce substantial visual loss
(C) are of shorter duration
(D) will not entail significant limb spasticity
(E) produce no sexual dysfunction

314. The evoked response pattern most often abnormal in patients with early MS is the

(A) brainstem auditory evoked response (BAER)
(B) far-field somatosensory evoked response (SSER)
(C) visual evoked response (VER)
(D) Jolly test
(E) sensory nerve conduction

315. On briskly flexing the neck forward, the patient with MS may report

(A) dystonic posturing of the legs
(B) an electrical sensation radiating down the spine or into the legs
(C) bilateral wristdrops
(D) spontaneous evacuation of the bladder and bilateral extensor plantar responses
(E) rapidly evolving hemifacial pain

316. Cystometrographic analysis of bladder function in the patient with MS and paraparesis will reveal all the following EXCEPT

(A) premature emptying of the bladder
(B) poor voluntary control of bladder emptying
(C) abnormally large residual volume of urine
(D) small maximum bladder volume
(E) increased bladder tone

Demyelinating Disorders
Answers

305. The answer is C. *(Lechtenberg, Multiple Sclerosis, p 7.)* Approximately 250,000 people in the United States carry the diagnosis of multiple sclerosis (MS). Most of the affected persons live in northern states, but no state is exempt from reports of MS. Because there is no test to unequivocally establish the diagnosis, the exact number of active cases in the United States can be approximated only very roughly.

306. The answer is A. *(Lechtenberg, Multiple Sclerosis, pp 37–68.)* White matter disease does not typically produce seizures. Because the incidence of seizures in the general population is between 0.5 and 1.0 percent, the probability that some individuals with multiple sclerosis will have seizures is high, but seizures, regardless of the specific type, are not suggestive of demyelinating disease. A patient with MR evidence of demyelination and recurrent episodes suggestive of seizure activity may have a progressive disturbance of myelin formation, such as adrenal leukodystrophy, or a viral encephalitis, such as that associated with HIV or cytomegalovirus infection.

307. The answer is A. *(Adams, ed 4. pp 576–578.)* General paresis is a form of neurosyphilis. Direct invasion of the brain by *Treponema pallidum* causes substantial damage to both white and gray matter, but the disease is not specifically demyelinating. Cerebral changes include atrophy, ventricular enlargement, and granular ependymitis. The brain in advanced general paresis exhibits little inflammatory reaction to the invading organism.

308. The answer is D. *(Lechtenberg, Synopsis, p 61.)* Adrenoleukodystrophy, multiple sclerosis, subacute sclerosing panencephalitis (SSPE), progressive multifocal leukoencephalopathy (PML), and metachromatic leukodystrophy are all demyelinating diseases, but PML is the only one confidently linked to a virus. The specific strains of papovavirus most often implicated in PML are BK, JC, and SV40. The patients at risk for this often-lethal demyelinating process are those with lymphomas, leukemias, and AIDS. Patients on immunosuppressants face substantially less risk, but are at more risk than the general population.

309. The answer is B. *(Adams, ed 4. p 17.)* Myelin is predominantly lipid, and when it is stripped away in a demyelinated plaque, the water content of that bit of white matter changes substantially. The MR scan is especially sensitive to water content because it is detecting proton content. Water is much richer in protons than is lipid. The density of white matter changes imperceptibly if it is demyelinated, but large plaques may be evident on CT scanning if a double dose of contrast is given and the small change in the blood-brain barrier that occurs with the inflammation in MS plaques is observed. Dye leaks across the slightly disabled blood-brain barrier and accumulates transiently in areas of demyelination.

310. The answer is C. *(Lechtenberg, Multiple Sclerosis, pp 71–72.)* The IgG content of the CSF remains elevated even between acute exacerbations of the multiple sclerosis. The IgG has a distinctive kappa light chain composition. This immunoglobulin typically accounts for more than 15 percent of the total protein content in the CSF of the patient with multiple sclerosis.

311. The answer is E. *(Lechtenberg, Multiple Sclerosis, pp 71–72.)* Between 85 and 90 percent of patients with MS exhibit oligoclonal banding on electrophoretic studies of their CSF. This limited number of bands of excess immunoglobulin indicates that the species of IgG produced by the disease fall into a relatively small number of families. The proteins are not highly diverse, as would be the case with a polyclonal gammopathy.

312. The answer is B. *(Lechtenberg, Multiple Sclerosis, pp 69–79.)* Although the protein content of the CSF is usually abnormal in MS, the serum protein constituents are usually unremarkable. Visual evoked responses may provide early evidence of an optic neuritis in patients with MS. Somatosensory evoked potentials are also helpful in making the diagnosis of MS by revealing unsuspected spinal cord demyelination. Both MR and CT scanning may show the plaques of demyelination in the brain if the patient has MS. MR may even reveal plaques in the spinal cord.

313. The answer is C. *(Lechtenberg, Multiple Sclerosis, pp 85–88.)* Management of acute exacerbations with ACTH or steroids may shorten the duration of the exacerbation and reduce some focal pain, such as that associated with optic neuritis, but this therapy does not affect the long-term disability exhibited by the patient. None of the currently available treatments affects the disability that accrues in the MS patient. Patients with severe MS routinely exhibit sexual dysfunction, visual impairment, and spastic paraparesis.

314. The answer is C. *(Lechtenberg, Multiple Sclerosis, pp 74–75.)* Optic neuritis occurs early and often in many patients with MS. This involves inflammation and demyelination of the optic nerve and slows conduction along the optic nerve. Components of the visual evoked response may be slowed or even absent. That an evoked response is disturbed is not proof that the patient has MS. Any problem producing optic neuritis will disturb the VER. The Jolly test is an evoked response involving muscles. A peripheral nerve is shocked at 5 to 15 times per second and the pattern of action potentials elicited in the muscle innervated is recorded. Sensory nerve conduction studies also involve an evoked response to a shock with the resulting signal tracked in the sensory nerve stimulated. Muscle and peripheral nerve function is typically normal in patients with MS, unless they have an unrelated disease of the peripheral nervous system.

315. The answer is B. *(Lechtenberg, Multiple Sclerosis, pp 65–68.)* The peculiar sensory phenomenon in which the patient feels an electrical sensation radiating down the spine when the neck is passively flexed is called Lhermitte's sign and is believed to signify spinal cord disease. Patients with MS who have little more than optic atrophy and no evidence of spinal cord involvement may report the sensation. Dystonic posturing may also occur in patients with MS, but the posturing is usually spontaneous. A massive Babinski response may produce bladder evacuation and extensor plantar responses as well as involuntary leg withdrawal in these same patients. This type of reflex response is usually elicited by stimuli to the feet or legs, rather than by manipulation of the neck or spine.

316. The answer is C. *(Lechtenberg, Multiple Sclerosis, pp 52–54.)* If the MS patient has paraparesis, he or she will also often have a spastic bladder. There is little or no residual urine in the bladder after emptying because bladder contractility is good, but distensibility is poor. The bladder does not distend substantially because of corticospinal tract disease, which produces spasticity. The affected person usually complains of urgency or urinary incontinence.

Developmental and Hereditary Disorders

DIRECTIONS: Each question below contains five suggested responses. Select the **one best** response to each question.

317. All the following usually develop with abetalipoproteinemia EXCEPT

(A) peripheral neuropathy
(B) gait and limb ataxia
(C) deafness
(D) visual loss
(E) dysarthria

318. The peripheral blood smear with abetalipoproteinemia usually reveals

(A) sickling of red cells
(B) hypersegmented neutrophils
(C) acanthocytes
(D) macrocytes
(E) thrombocytopenia

319. A defect in neural tube closure indicates an injury to the nervous system during fetal development

(A) between 30 and 40 weeks
(B) between 20 and 30 weeks
(C) between 10 and 20 weeks
(D) between 5 and 10 weeks
(E) before 5 weeks

320. With Sturge-Weber syndrome, a port-wine stain (nevus flammeus) usually extends

(A) from the base of the neck to the angle of the jaw
(B) over both sides of the face
(C) over one side of the face
(D) over the distribution of V3
(E) over the distribution of V3 and C2

321. The intracranial calcifications typical of Sturge-Weber syndrome are in the

(A) arachnoid
(B) pia mater
(C) dura mater
(D) subarachnoid space
(E) cerebral cortex

322. With phenylketonuria (PKU), serum may exhibit dangerously high levels of

(A) creatine kinase
(B) nicotinamide
(C) phenylketone
(D) lactate dehydrogenase
(E) phenylalanine

323. Hartnup disease is a hereditary disorder causing gait difficulty, emotional lability, delusions, and tremor that may respond to large supplementary doses of

(A) tryptophan
(B) nicotinamide
(C) thiamine
(D) pyridoxine
(E) alpha-tocopherol

324. Hepatosplenomegaly is most likely with

(A) Tay-Sachs disease
(B) Niemann-Pick disease
(C) Alpers disease
(D) subacute necrotizing encephalopathy
(E) Wilson disease (hepatolenticular degeneration)

325. Anencephaly is probably most often related to maternal

(A) age
(B) multiparity
(C) infection
(D) nutrition
(E) epilepsy

326. All the following have been found to be associated with defects in neural tube closure EXCEPT

(A) maternal hyperthermia
(B) irradiation
(C) penicillin G
(D) salicylates
(E) antimetabolites

327. With agenesis of the corpus callosum, the MR scan will reveal

(A) atrophy of the frontal lobes
(B) abnormally shaped lateral and third ventricles
(C) cerebellar aplasia
(D) schizencephaly
(E) encephaloclastic porencephaly

328. With metachromatic leukodystrophy, the hereditary enzymatic defect is in

(A) hexosaminidase A
(B) hexosaminidase B
(C) glucocerebrosidase
(D) arylsulfatase A
(E) phosphofructokinase

329. The diagnosis of metachromatic leukodystrophy can usually be made on the basis of

(A) MR scanning
(B) nerve biopsy
(C) red blood cell morphology
(D) CSF cell morphology
(E) EEG

330. Canavan disease is a type of leukodystrophy in which infants may exhibit

(A) precocious puberty
(B) hydrocephalus
(C) macrocephaly
(D) neonatal seizures
(E) choreoathetosis

331. Ferruginous deposits in the basal ganglia of the brain are seen with Hallervorden-Spatz disease and

(A) Pelizaeus-Merzbacher disease
(B) Huntington disease
(C) sex-linked adrenoleukodystrophy
(D) autosomal dominant adrenoleukodystrophy
(E) Sydenham chorea

332. In neuronal ceroid lipofuscinosis, the accumulating material typical of this metabolic disease is evident on

(A) MR scanning
(B) CT scanning
(C) urinalysis
(D) CSF examination
(E) brain biopsy

333. The most common cause of hereditary mental retardation in men is

(A) Turner syndrome
(B) Klinefelter syndrome
(C) fragile X syndrome
(D) Reye syndrome
(E) tuberous sclerosis

334. Women carrying fragile X chromosomes

(A) are invariably normal
(B) have mild retardation in about one-third of cases
(C) have high arched palates and hypotelorism
(D) have hyperextensible joints
(E) have prominent thumbs

335. A 40-year-old man with polycystic liver disease and retinal angiomas acutely developed headache and progressive obtundation. Within 2 h he had evidence of tonsillar herniation and died. The most likely explanation for his catastrophic deterioration is

(A) intracerebral hemorrhage
(B) intrathalamic hemorrhage
(C) intraventricular hemorrhage
(D) subarachnoid hemorrhage
(E) intracerebellar hemorrhage

336. All the following are characteristic of the von Hippel-Lindau syndrome EXCEPT

(A) pancreatic cysts
(B) hydrocephalus
(C) epididymal cysts
(D) erythrocytosis
(E) splenic cysts

337. Aqueductal stenosis may develop as a consequence of

(A) phenytoin exposure
(B) intrauterine infection
(C) status epilepticus
(D) protracted migraine
(E) intervertebral disk herniation

338. Arachnoid cysts in the head usually produce

(A) no symptoms
(B) epilepsy
(C) dementia
(D) hemiparesis
(E) anosmia

339. Subungual fibromas develop in as many as one out of five persons with

(A) tuberous sclerosis
(B) Tay-Sachs disease
(C) galactosemia
(D) Sturge-Weber syndrome
(E) ataxia telangiectasia

340. A 50-year-old man complaining of dizziness is found to have a cyst occupying 50 percent of his posterior fossa and incomplete fusion of the cerebellar elements inferiorly. There is no evidence of an obstructive hydrocephalus. His longevity can be estimated to be

(A) less than 3 months
(B) less than 1 year
(C) less than 5 years
(D) less than 10 years
(E) unaffected by this finding

341. All the following are often associated with a Dandy-Walker malformation EXCEPT

(A) dysgenesis of the vermis
(B) herniation of the cerebellar tonsils
(C) high tentorium cerebelli
(D) elevation of the transverse sinuses
(E) enlarged posterior fossa

342. Other than the brain, organs frequently exhibiting abnormalities in persons with Dandy-Walker malformations include the

(A) kidneys
(B) heart
(C) lungs
(D) intestines
(E) liver

343. A relatively common defect associated with the posterior fossa anomalies of the Arnold-Chiari (type 2 Chiari) malformation is

(A) a renal cyst
(B) pulmonary atelectasis
(C) spina bifida
(D) holoprosencephaly
(E) a hepatic cyst

344. All the following are characteristic of the Arnold-Chiari malformation EXCEPT

(A) an enlarged posterior fossa
(B) a caudally displaced medulla oblongata
(C) a caudally displaced cerebellar vermis
(D) a low tentorium cerebelli
(E) an elongated fourth ventricle

345. The most common skin lesion developing with tuberous sclerosis is

(A) café au lait spots
(B) port-wine nevus
(C) adenoma sebaceum
(D) shagreen patches
(E) senile keratosis

346. Tuberous sclerosis is inherited in

(A) a sex-linked recessive pattern
(B) an autosomal dominant pattern
(C) an autosomal recessive pattern
(D) a pattern most consistent with newly arising mutations
(E) a pattern suggesting a mitochrondrial gene defect

347. Retinal problems with tuberous sclerosis

(A) include retinal phakomas
(B) include retinitis pigmentosa
(C) include retinal telangiectasias
(D) include retinoblastomas
(E) are generally not part of the disease

348. Infantile spasms occur in what percentage of children with tuberous sclerosis?

(A) 1
(B) 15
(C) 40
(D) 75
(E) 100

349. The treatment of choice for children with infantile spasms is

(A) carbamazepine (Tegretol)
(B) phenobarbital
(C) phenytoin (Dilantin)
(D) divalproex sodium (Depakote)
(E) adrenocorticotropic hormone (ACTH)

350. What percentage of patients with tuberous sclerosis have mental retardation?

(A) 1
(B) 25
(C) 45
(D) 65
(E) 85

351. Calcifications evident on the skull x-ray or CT scan of a patient with tuberous sclerosis usually represent

(A) calcified subependymal glial nodules
(B) calcified meningeal adhesions
(C) meningeal psammoma bodies
(D) calcified astrocytomas
(E) calcified granulomas

352. Flank pain acutely developing in a person with tuberous sclerosis is likely to be from

(A) renal calculi
(B) hemorrhage into a renal cyst
(C) hemorrhage into a renal tumor
(D) embolic infarction of renal tissue
(E) ureteral obstruction

353. Pulmonary cystic disease usually appears with tuberous sclerosis

(A) in the newborn
(B) during childhood
(C) at puberty
(D) toward the end of adolescence
(E) during adult life

354. Café au lait spots are areas of hyperpigmented skin commonly found on patients with

(A) tuberous sclerosis
(B) neurofibromatosis
(C) multiple sclerosis
(D) Sturge-Weber syndrome
(E) ataxia telangiectasia

355. Maternal factors worth considering in the investigation of neonatal seizures include all the following EXCEPT

(A) illnesses during pregnancy
(B) maternal drug use
(C) familial histories of seizure
(D) maternal head trauma
(E) maternal skin lesions

356. Congenital abnormalities associated with fetal exposure to phenytoin and other antiepileptic medications include all the following EXCEPT

(A) ventricular septal defects
(B) nail hypoplasia
(C) cataracts
(D) cleft palate
(E) hip dysplasia

357. The newborn infant with motor neuron disease is likely to exhibit

(A) seizures
(B) hypotonia
(C) hypsarrhythmia
(D) Moro reflexes
(E) spina bifida

358. The enzymatic defect responsible for Tay-Sachs disease is in

(A) hexosaminidase A
(B) hexosaminidase B
(C) glucocerebrosidase
(D) sphingomyelinase
(E) beta-galactosidase

359. Common clinical signs of Tay-Sachs disease include all the following EXCEPT

(A) abnormal startle response
(B) delayed psychomotor development
(C) microcephaly
(D) axial hypotonia
(E) spasticity

360. Many of the children with Tay-Sachs disease develop blindness before they die, with retinal accumulation of gangliosides that produces

(A) optic neuritis
(B) cherry-red spots
(C) chorioretinitis
(D) retinal detachments
(E) waxy exudates

361. All the following typically occur in Tay-Sachs disease EXCEPT

(A) hyperacusis
(B) optic atrophy
(C) cerebellar atrophy
(D) G_{M2} ganglioside accumulation in the brain
(E) hepatosplenomegaly

362. Cerebral palsy (CP) is a static encephalopathy because

(A) deficits do not appear after birth
(B) the injury to the brain does not progress
(C) affected persons fail to reach any developmental milestones on time
(D) affected persons have resting tremors
(E) the EEG exhibits a disorganized background rhythm

363. All the following are possible areas of impairment associated with cerebral palsy (CP) EXCEPT

(A) cognition
(B) language
(C) sensation
(D) vision
(E) digestion

364. The brain of the patient with Down syndrome (trisomy 21) is typically

(A) smaller than normal for age and body size
(B) larger than normal for age and body size
(C) abnormally long in anteroposterior measurements
(D) hydrocephalic
(E) excessively convoluted

365. Porencephaly usually develops as a consequence of

(A) fetal alcohol syndrome
(B) vascular or other destructive injuries to the fetal brain
(C) trisomy 13
(D) trisomy 21
(E) the Dandy-Walker syndrome

DIRECTIONS: The group of questions below consists of four lettered headings followed by a set of numbered items. For each numbered item select

A	if the item is associated with	(A) **only**
B	if the item is associated with	(B) **only**
C	if the item is associated with	**both** (A) and (B)
D	if the item is associated with	**neither** (A) nor (B)

Each lettered heading may be used **once, more than once, or not at all.**

Questions 366–369

(A) Mental retardation
(B) Microcephaly
(C) Both
(D) Neither

366. Uncorrected congenital hydrocephalus

367. Fetal alcohol syndrome

368. Adult Chiari (type 1) malformation

369. Prenatal cytomegalovirus infection

Developmental and Hereditary Disorders

Answers

317. The answer is C. *(Gilman, Disorders, p 242.)* Abetalipoproteinemia (Bassen-Kornzweig syndrome) usually becomes symptomatic during childhood with the initial complaints most often mimicking Friedreich disease, a hereditary ataxia. Position sense is lost and extensor plantar responses develop as the disease progresses. As is true for Friedreich disease, dementia is not an obvious part of the syndrome. Neuropathy, gait ataxia, limb dysmetria, visual acuity deterioration, and dysarthria may become severe in the patient with abetalipoproteinemia as the disease progresses over the course of years.

318. The answer is C. *(Gilman, Disorders, p 242.)* Acanthocytes are spiked or crenated red blood cells. These are an unusual hematologic finding in patients with ataxia and are often diagnostic of abetalipoproteinemia (Bassen-Kornzweig syndrome). Autopsy examination of the CNS in patients with abetalipoproteinemia reveals posterior column and spinocerebellar tract degeneration.

319. The answer is E. *(Davis, p 185.)* The fusion of the lateral elements of the neural fold on the embryo starts at 22 days of gestation. The anterior pore closes first at about 24 days and the posterior neuropore should close at 26 to 28 days. For a toxin to produce a defect in neural tube closure, it must exert its effect during the first month of fetal development.

320. The answer is C. *(Davis, pp 234–235.)* The nevus associated with Sturge-Weber syndrome invariably extends over the sensory distribution of V1, the first division of the trigeminal nerve. The lesion usually stays to one side of the face. Affected persons will usually also have an angioma of the choroid of the eye.

321. The answer is E. *(Davis, p 235.)* Calcium is deposited in the brain of the patient with Sturge-Weber syndrome presumably because the abnormal vessels overlying the brain allow calcium, as well as iron, across the defective blood-brain barrier. The calcifications follow the gyral pattern of the cortex in which they form and produce a picture on plain skull roentgenograms often called "railroad tracking." The cerebral lesions are usually, but not always, on the same side as the facial nevus.

322. The answer is E. *(Adams, ed 4. pp 790–792.)* PKU is inherited as an autosomal recessive trait. It occurs in at least two forms. In one form, intolerance of phenylalanine is extreme, and dietary intake of that amino acid must be restricted from birth. Alternatively, some persons have hyperphenylalaninemia without phenylketonuria. This latter group does not suffer the CNS damage seen with in utero exposure to high phenylalanine levels. Such in utero exposure will occur if the mother is homozygous for PKU. If the mother is normal, infants with PKU are born with essentially normal nervous systems. Damage develops after birth in the susceptible group as serum phenylalanine levels rise.

323. The answer is B. *(Adams, ed 4. pp 793–842.)* With Hartnup disease there is intestinal malabsorption of tryptophan and other neutral amino acids. Tryptophan serves as a precursor for nicotinamide, but with more than 400 mg of nicotinamide daily, the tryptophan malabsorption becomes less problematic. Excess tryptophan does not help the patient, presumably because tryptophan transport across the intestinal wall plateaus at a low level. Inheritance appears to be autosomal recessive. Affected children develop a scaly erythematous rash on the face similar to that seen with pellagra. The ataxia exhibited by the affected children may be episodic.

324. The answer is B. *(Adams, ed 4. p 784.)* Niemann-Pick disease is inherited as an autosomal recessive trait. By 9 months of age patients with the infantile form usually have prominent hepatosplenomegaly. A deficiency of sphingomyelinase in hepatocytes is diagnostic for the disease.

325. The answer is D. *(Davis, p 186.)* The only factor that appears to correlate with the probability of having a child with anencephaly is socioeconomic status. This suggests that nutrition plays a role in the development of an anencephalic fetus. Both anencephaly and myelomeningoceles may be suggested prenatally by elevated maternal serum alpha-fetoprotein levels.

326. The answer is C. *(Davis, p 187.)* Many agents have been linked to problems with neural tube formation or closure, but none causes problems in a large segment of the population. Colchicine, papaverine, and caffeine, as well as irradiation, hyperthermia, antimetabolites, and salicylates, may increase the risk of neural tube malformations. The vitamin most clearly implicated in cases involving hypervitaminosis is vitamin A. Some antiepileptic drugs have been associated with an increased incidence of defects in neural tube closure, but congenital malformations as a group are slightly increased in epileptic persons even if they are not taking antiepileptic drugs before or during the pregnancy. Divalproex sodium is the antiepileptic most clearly linked to defects in neural tube closure, but even with this drug the incidence of spina bifida, meningoceles, myelomeningoceles, and other consequences of failed neural tube closure is small.

327. The answer is B. *(Davis, p 200.)* On coronal sections of the brain, the lateral ventricles will have a typical "bat-wing" conformation if the patient has agenesis of the corpus callosum. The third ventricle may be dilated and open onto the surface of the brain. Patients with this congenital anomaly may be asymptomatic or may exhibit a variety of cognitive disorders. In the Aicardi syndrome, agenesis of the corpus callosum is associated with retardation, epilepsy, vertebral anomalies, and chorioretinitis.

328. The answer is D. *(Lechtenberg, Synopsis, p 152.)* The enzymatic defect in metachromatic leukodystrophy is transmitted in an autosomal recessive fashion. The affected person usually has retardation, ataxia, spasticity, and sensory disturbances, but individual elements of this disorder may appear alone in less serious cases. Patients with metachromatic leukodystrophy usually develop symptoms during infancy. Those first problems often involve gait and ocular motor problems.

329. The answer is B. *(Lechtenberg, Synopsis, p 152.)* Sulfatide granules may be evident in nerve tissue, as well as in tissue outside the nervous system, in persons with metachromatic leukodystrophy. The disease is usually fatal within a few years of obvious symptoms. At autopsy, there may be evidence of dysmyelination or demyelination in the CNS, as well as in the peripheral nervous system.

330. The answer is C. *(Lechtenberg, Synopsis, p 152.)* That something is wrong with the infant with Canavan disease, a type of leukodystrophy, is usually evident soon after birth. Even if macrocephaly is not prominent, the child will usually exhibit hypotonia. *N*-acetylaspartic acid can be detected in the urine of these children. Optic atrophy, intellectual decline, and death usually ensue within the first few years of life.

331. The answer is A. *(Lechtenberg, Synopsis, p 152.)* Pelizaeus-Merzbacher disease is a type of leukodystrophy with many of the features exhibited in Canavan disease. Unlike Canavan disease, the affected children usually develop marked spasticity rather than hypotonia. The disease appears later than Canavan disease and progresses more slowly. It does, however, usually result in death during childhood.

332. The answer is E. *(Lechtenberg, Synopsis, pp 152–153.)* The typical intracellular inclusions characteristic of neuronal ceroid lipofuscinosis, a hereditary neurodegenerative disorder, are usually evident on brain or nerve biopsy. The metabolic defect underlying neuronal ceroid lipofuscinosis is unknown. Affected persons may develop ataxia, dementia, and seizures as the disease progresses. Different forms of this disease characteristically begin at different times of life, with infantile, juvenile, and adult forms being most commonly reported.

333. The answer is C. *(Lechtenberg, Synopsis, p 153.)* With the fragile X syndrome, the terminal elements of the long arm of the abnormal X chromosome appear stretched or broken away from the rest of the chromosome. Retardation usually becomes evident during childhood. Affected men have large ears, a high arched palate, hypotelorism, and large testes.

334. The answer is B. *(Lechtenberg, Synopsis, p 153.)* Men with the fragile X syndrome have hyperextensible joints and prominent thumbs, but carrier women may appear quite normal. The abnormal chromosome may be detected in fetal lymphocytes and fibroblasts, thereby allowing for prenatal screening. Epilepsy develops in many affected persons, but the seizures are usually easily controlled, unlike the case with other hereditary causes of epilepsy.

335. The answer is E. *(Gilman, Disorders, pp 280–283.)* Polycystic liver disease, retinal angiomata, and hemorrhage-prone cerebellar tumors are the hallmarks of the von Hippel–Lindau syndrome. This is an autosomal dominant inherited disorder with variable penetrance. Men are more commonly affected than women. Persons with this disorder usually die from intracerebellar hemorrhages or metastatic renal carcinoma.

336. The answer is B. *(Gilman, Disorders, pp 280–283.)* Although cysts may develop in the cerebellum in persons with the von Hippel–Lindau syndrome, these usually do not become sufficiently large to cause an obstructive hydrocephalus. Other abnormalities occurring with this syndrome include adenomas in many organs. Hemangiomas may be evident in the bones, adrenals, and ovaries. Hemangioblastomas may develop in the spinal cord or brainstem, as well as in the cerebellum. These hemangioblastomas often bleed and produce potentially lethal intracranial hematomas. Patients who survive these hemorrhagic tumors often develop renal carcinomas later in life and succumb to this complication of the syndrome.

337. The answer is B. *(Davis, p 224.)* The aqueduct of Sylvius may be narrowed or completely obstructed after a fetal encephalitis. The most likely agents are viruses, such as mumps. If the stenosis is extreme or obstruction is complete, the child may be born with hydrocephalus.

338. The answer is A. *(Davis, pp 228–229.)* Arachnoid cysts are congenital anomalies that may produce hydrocephalus if they are large and develop at the incisura of the tentorium cerebelli. Occasionally they do imitate tumors, but they are not neoplastic lesions. They develop as malformations of the meninges, and most commonly occur in the sylvian fissure.

339. The answer is A. *(Johnson, ed 3. p 108.)* Subungual fibromas are benign tumors developing under the fingernails or toenails. They may develop alone or in association with other tumors, such as those arising in the brain or kidneys. They are not considered sufficient for the diagnosis of tuberous sclerosis, but often develop in persons with this hereditary disturbance of CNS development.

340. The answer is E. *(Gilman, Disorders, pp 264–265.)* That the cerebellar elements are not fused in the midline suggests an asymptomatic Dandy-Walker malformation. This congenital disorder of brain formation may become symptomatic soon after birth if an obstructive hydrocephalus develops as one facet of the anomaly. In the absence of an obstructive hydrocephalus, the patient may remain asymptomatic throughout life.

341. The answer is B. *(Gilman, Disorders, pp 265–278.)* The cerebellar tonsils are herniated through the foramen magnum in the adult Chiari (type 1) malformation. The cerebellar tonsils with a Dandy-Walker malformation are unrecognizable or lie abnormally high in the posterior fossa. Both the Dandy-Walker and Chiari malformations involve abnormal development of the entire posterior fossa and adjacent structures.

342. The answer is A. *(Gilman, Disorders, pp 264–269.)* Patients with the Dandy-Walker malformation commonly exhibit a renal anomaly. This anomaly is usually innocuous and may consist of nothing more than a renal malformation. Other congenital malformations in these patients include polydactyly, cleft palate, and spinal dysplasia. In the CNS, agenesis of the corpus callosum and gyral anomalies in the cerebrum are relatively common.

343. The answer is C. (*Gilman, Disorders, pp 272–278.*) Spina bifida may be extreme in some of the children affected by the Arnold-Chiari (Chiari type 2) malformation. A myelomeningocele may be present at the level of the spina bifida. Spinal cord tissues may extend into this mass and lie just under the skin covering the neural tube defect. Children with obvious spinal defects usually have persistent problems with leg movements and bladder and bowel control.

344. The answer is A. (*Gilman, Disorders, p 276.*) The posterior fossa is abnormally small in persons with Arnold-Chiari malformation. Other features obvious in the posterior fossa include a beaked cervicomedullary junction, a conical (rather than quadrigeminal) tectal plate, and aqueductal stenosis. Other elements of the brain are variably deformed. Even the cerebrum may exhibit microgyria.

345. The answer is C. (*Johnson, ed 3. pp 108–110.*) Both shagreen patches and adenoma sebaceum occur with tuberous sclerosis, but adenoma sebaceum occurs in about 90 percent of patients and shagreen patches occur in only about 20 percent. Adenoma sebaceum usually becomes apparent on the face between 2 and 5 years of age. These skin lesions may develop into difficult-to-treat angiofibromas of the skin.

346. The answer is B. (*Johnson, ed 3. p 108.*) Although the inheritance pattern of tuberous sclerosis is autosomal dominant, the penetrance is variable. A severely impaired child may be born to a negligibly affected parent. Despite the consensus that inheritance is autosomally dominant, estimates of spontaneous mutations in affected persons are as high as 70 percent.

347. The answer is A. (*Johnson, ed 3. pp 108–110.*) Retinal phakomas, which require no treatment, are a principal criterion for making the diagnosis of tuberous sclerosis, and along with adenoma sebaceum and periventricular tubers, they are virtually pathognomonic. Other findings typical of tuberous sclerosis include ash leaf spots, shagreen patches, CNS calcifications, renal tumors, cardiac rhabdomyomas, and seizure disorders.

348. The answer is C. (*Johnson, ed 3. p 108.*) Seizures of some type occur in more than 40 percent of persons with tuberous sclerosis, and at least 40 percent have infantile spasms during the first years of life. All those who have tuberous sclerosis and mental retardation have seizures. Only about 70 percent of those with normal intelligence have seizures. Seizure types include infantile spasms, complex partial seizures, and generalized tonic-clonic seizures.

349. The answer is E. *(Johnson, ed 3. pp 108–109.)* ACTH is usually given as a gel intramuscularly to control infantile spasms in children with tuberous sclerosis. Forty to 80 mg is divided into two doses. Treatment continues until the infantile spasms abate or the EEG pattern of hypsarrhythmia resolves. This usually requires 6 to 8 weeks of treatment. The ACTH should not be stopped abruptly.

350. The answer is D. *(Johnson, ed 3. p 109.)* Of the 65 percent of patients with tuberous sclerosis who are retarded, half are severely retarded. Seizures are invariably associated with retardation. About 20 percent of patients with tuberous sclerosis develop the Lennox-Gastaut syndrome with persistent seizures and significant mental retardation. These children usually have a mixed seizure disorder, whereas those without Lennox-Gastaut syndrome most often have complex partial seizures.

351. The answer is A. *(Johnson, ed 3. p 109.)* By 5 years of age, more than half the patients with tuberous sclerosis will have subependymal glial nodules that have calcified. These nodules usually do not become malignant, but they may enlarge sufficiently to produce an obstructive hydrocephalus. Ventriculo-peritoneal shunting may be needed if obstruction develops.

352. The answer is C. *(Johnson, ed 3. p 110.)* Angiomyolipomas commonly develop in the kidneys of persons with tuberous sclerosis. They are benign tumors and often develop bilaterally. About 10 percent of patients with this tumor develop massive hemorrhaging into the tumor. Tumors larger than 4 cm are generally considered at risk for this type of catastrophe and should be removed or embolized prophylactically.

353. The answer is E. *(Johnson, ed 3. p 109.)* Pulmonary cysts typically appear during the third and fourth decades of life in persons with tuberous sclerosis. Women have these lesions more often than men, but women typically survive longer with tuberous sclerosis because they are much less neurologically impaired than the affected men. These pulmonic cysts may become symptomatic with signs of cor pulmonale or pneumothorax.

354. The answer is B. *(Johnson, ed 3. pp 101–108.)* Café au lait spots in patients with neurofibromatosis are usually larger than a few centimeters and occur in several locations in individual patients. Some have ragged edges and are called coast of Maine spots. They occur with both type 1 and type 2 neurofibromatosis, but are much more common with type 1.

355. The answer is D. *(Johnson, ed 3. pp 24–25.)* Even if a pregnant woman experiences sufficient head trauma to produce seizures that recur, the occurrence of posttraumatic seizures in the parent does not increase the risk of seizures in the newborn. Skin lesions on the parent associated with seizures in the infant may, however, indicate that a hereditary neurocutaneous disorder, such as tuberous sclerosis or neurofibromatosis, is responsible for the child's seizure disorder. Alternatively, maternal illnesses during the pregnancy may support the hypothesis that an intrauterine infection is responsible for the child's seizures. Prescription or nonprescription drug use during pregnancy may make the neonate susceptible to withdrawal seizures.

356. The answer is C. *(Lechtenberg, Seizure, pp 180–185.)* All the widely used antiepileptic medications increase the risk of birth defects in the offspring of women taking the drugs, but the teratogenicity of phenytoin, carbamazepine, and divalproex sodium is slight. Ocular defects are not typical effects of any of these drugs, but skeletal and cardiac anomalies do occur. Most epileptologists believe that carbamazepine has the lowest teratogenicity of the commonly used antiepileptics.

357. The answer is B. *(Lechtenberg, Synopsis, p 101.)* The child with congenital weakness, hypotonia, and muscle atrophy may have Werdnig-Hoffman disease, a congenital motor neuron disease. This is an especially lethal form of motor neuron disease and may limit the child's life expectancy to weeks or months. A similar pattern of disease appearing in older children is less lethal and is called Kugelberg-Welander disease. These types of motor neuron diseases are also known as spinal muscular atrophies. Anterior horn cell disease is presumed to be a pivotal feature of diseases in this category.

358. The answer is A. *(Adams, ed 4. p 783.)* Tay-Sachs disease is inherited in an autosomally recessive pattern. Death usually occurs by 3 to 5 years of age. The enzymatic defect in hexosaminidase A allows the accumulation of gangliosides. Fibroblasts collected during amniocentesis may be cultured and checked for the enzyme defect to allow diagnosis of the disorder prenatally.

359. The answer is C. *(Adams, ed 4. p 783.)* Macrocephaly, rather than microcephaly, may develop as Tay-Sachs disease progresses. Some children with Tay-Sachs disease do have microcephaly initially, but this is an unreliable clinical sign of the disease. Affected infants may show regression and loss of psychomotor milestones if development has been progressive for several months. Prominent signs of corticospinal tract disease usually evolve after the appearance of axial hypotonia.

360. The answer is B. *(Adams, ed 4. p 783.)* More than 90 percent of children with Tay-Sachs disease develop cherry-red spots on the retina. The red spot at the fovea develops as retinal ganglion cells become distended with glycolipid. There are no ganglion cell bodies overlying the fovea, and so the red color of the vascular choroid is apparent in this region but obscured by more opaque glycolipid-engorged cells over the remainder of the retina.

361. The answer is E. *(Davis, pp 299–300.)* Ganglioside levels with Tay-Sachs disease may be elevated in visceral tissue, but the liver and spleen do not exhibit the enlargement typical of other lipidoses. Affected infants are usually normal at birth, but an exaggerated startle response by a few months of age usually points to the development of hyperacusis. Hypotonia may develop, but it is invariably followed by the appearance of corticospinal tract signs, including spasticity.

362. The answer is B. *(Johnson, ed 3. p 92.)* A static encephalopathy is one in which brain damage has been arrested but neurologic problems persist. Establishing that the brain lesion is not progressive may require extensive testing. A newborn with a static encephalopathy is said to have cerebral palsy (CP). Neurodegenerative diseases with slow or stepwise progressions may appear to be static encephalopathies over the course of months, but prove to be progressive encephalopathies over the course of years. The brain lesion with CP is static, but the deficits associated with CP may evolve as the child matures.

363. The answer is E. *(Johnson, ed 3. p 93.)* Although CP is a neurologic disturbance and all the problems associated with it should be traceable to CNS damage, the alimentary tract may be disturbed. Digestion per se is not impaired, but affected children often exhibit esophageal reflux or aspiration. Because of the CNS damage, feeding may be a problem for these children and malnutrition may develop.

364. The answer is A. *(Davis, p 182.)* The brain of the patient with Down syndrome is typically foreshortened. The gyral pattern is simplified, and the frontal lobes are small. The occipital lobes may be slanted, and the overall shape of the skull is abnormal.

365. The answer is B. *(Davis, pp 183–184.)* In utero damage to the fetal brain may be evident at birth as large cysts in the brain. One or more of these intracerebral cysts is called *porencephaly.* Some pathologists believe that a related abnormality, *schizencephaly,* in which brain segmentation is abnormal, is caused by similar phenomena. These phenomena would include incidents such as strokes and viral encephalitides in the fetal brain.

366–369. The answers are: 366-A, 367-C, 368-D, 369-C. *(Adams, ed 4. pp 506–507, 884–885. Gilman, Disorders, pp 269–278. Lechtenberg, AIDS, pp 113–114.)* A variety of conditions will produce congenital hydrocephalus, and any condition producing apparent hydrocephalus at birth may produce mental retardation. Correction of the hydrocephalus at or soon after birth reduces the probability of retardation as a direct effect of the hydrocephalus, but conditions that cause damage to the brain as well as obstruct the flow of CSF may leave the patient retarded. If the hydrocephalus is not corrected, pressure on the cerebral cortex will produce retardation and ultimately death. An uncorrected hydrocephalus may not be lethal for many years. The pressure buildup within the skull of the newborn causes macrocephaly rather than microcephaly.

Mental retardation and microcephaly are the most common neurologic consequences of fetal alcohol syndrome. How alcohol produces the various neurologic problems characteristic of the fetal alcohol syndrome is unknown, but most evidence suggests that alcohol exerts a direct toxic effect. The fetus appears to be most susceptible to the teratogenic effects of alcohol between the fourth and sixth months of development.

Chiari malformations are primarily abnormalities of hindbrain development. With the type 1 abnormality, the cerebellar tonsils extend below the foramen magnum. With the type 2, cerebellar anatomy is usually much more deranged, and the cerebellar vermis lies well below the foramen magnum. The type 2 malformations most often become symptomatic at birth or during infancy and may produce hydrocephalus with retardation, but the adult or type 1 malformations appear in the fourth or fifth decades of life without any associated retardation. Neither type of malformation is likely to cause microcephaly.

Neurologic problems developing in the infant with a prenatal cytomegalovirus (CMV) infection include retardation, microcephaly, seizures, and hearing deficits. The virus often causes chorioretinitis, optic atrophy, and architectural changes throughout the brain. The cerebellum in the affected infant may be atrophic, and focal accumulations of microglial cells, called *microglial nodules,* may be prominent throughout much of the brain.

Neuromuscular Disorders

DIRECTIONS: Each question below contains five suggested responses. Select the **one best** response to each question.

370. Dermatomyositis in the patient over 60 years of age is associated with a higher-than-expected incidence of neoplasms in all the following organs EXCEPT

(A) brain
(B) lung
(C) breast
(D) ovary
(E) intestinal tract

371. Electromyographic studies of patients with polymyositis will characteristically reveal all the following EXCEPT

(A) increased insertional activity
(B) fibrillations
(C) positive sharp waves
(D) fasciculations
(E) polyphasic, low-amplitude motor unit potentials

372. The most obvious site of disease in myasthenia gravis is the

(A) anterior horn cell
(B) neuromuscular junction
(C) sensory ganglion
(D) parasympathetic ganglia
(E) sympathetic chain

373. The most common manifestation of muscle weakness with myasthenia gravis is

(A) diaphragmatic weakness
(B) wristdrop
(C) ocular muscle weakness
(D) footdrop
(E) dysphagia

374. Inflammatory muscle disease characterized by noncaseating granulomas may have been caused by

(A) cysticercosis
(B) tuberculosis
(C) sarcoidosis
(D) schistosomiasis
(E) carcinomatosis

375. The association of a heliotrope rash with myopathy suggests

(A) histiocytosis X
(B) dermatomyositis
(C) myasthenia gravis
(D) thymoma
(E) tuberous sclerosis

376. Any of the following may cause a myopathy EXCEPT

(A) giant cell arteritis
(B) hyperthyroidism
(C) scleroderma
(D) phosphofructokinase deficiency
(E) herpes simplex

377. Duchenne dystrophy is a sex-linked disorder involving the gene responsible for the synthesis of

(A) glucose-6-phosphatase
(B) hexosaminidase B
(C) myosin
(D) dystrophin
(E) actin

378. Duchenne dystrophy affects approximately

(A) 1 in 3000 infants
(B) 1 in 3000 male infants
(C) 1 in 30,000 infants
(D) 1 in 30,000 male infants
(E) 1 in 50,000 infants

379. For a girl to have Duchenne dystrophy, she must have

(A) Turner syndrome (XO)
(B) Klinefelter syndrome (XXY)
(C) two affected parents
(D) an affected father
(E) an affected brother

380. With Duchenne dystrophy, pseudohypertrophy routinely

(A) does not occur
(B) is limited to the shoulder girdle
(C) is limited to the hip girdle
(D) is limited to the calf muscles
(E) is limited to the thigh muscles

381. The spontaneous mutation rate for the dystrophin gene is presumed to be high because

(A) men with Duchenne dystrophy do not reproduce
(B) the incidence of Duchenne dystrophy is increasing
(C) numerous birth defects occur in families with Duchenne dystrophy
(D) men may become symptomatic after adolescence
(E) genetic studies of eggs in human ovaries reveal an excess of abnormal dystrophin genes

382. Intellectual function in children with Duchenne dystrophy is usually

(A) markedly impaired
(B) slightly impaired
(C) normal
(D) slightly better than the general population
(E) markedly superior to the general population

383. A woman carrying the gene for Duchenne dystrophy may exhibit substantial elevations in her serum

(A) ammonia
(B) myoglobin
(C) phosphofructokinase
(D) creatine kinase
(E) hexosaminidase

384. Biopsy of muscles in persons with Duchenne dystrophy may reveal all the following EXCEPT

(A) excessive variation in the diameter of muscle fibers
(B) infiltration of fat between muscle fibers
(C) excessive connective tissue where muscle fibers would normally appear
(D) enlargement of muscle fibers
(E) ragged red fibers

385. A 37-year-old man complained of difficulty relaxing his grip on his golf club after putting. He also complained of problems with excessive somnolence. Examination revealed early cataract development, testicular atrophy, and baldness. His family noted that he had become increasingly stubborn and hostile over the past 3 years. His electrocardiogram (ECG) revealed a minor conduction defect. An electromyogram (EMG) of this man will probably reveal

(A) repetitive discharges with minor stimulation
(B) polyphasic giant action potentials
(C) fasciculations
(D) fibrillations
(E) positive waves

Neuromuscular Disorders

Answers

370. The answer is A. *(Johnson, ed 3. pp 403–404.)* In dermatomyositis, an inflammatory myopathy is associated with a typical rash. The most common components of this rash are the violaceous discoloration developing around the eyes and the erythema developing over the knuckles. Because of the higher probability of malignancy in adults with dermatomyositis, patients diagnosed with this inflammatory disease should routinely undergo a variety of diagnostic studies. These studies include rectal and breast examinations, periodic screens for occult blood in the stool, and hemograms. Sputum cytologies and chest x-rays, as well as urine cytologic studies, are recommended by some physicians.

371. The answer is D. *(Johnson, ed 3. p 403.)* Polymyositis is an inflammatory disease of muscle. Fasciculations are characteristic of anterior horn cell disease, which is unrelated to polymyositis. The EMG changes occurring with polymyositis are usually more prominent in the proximal than in the distal limb muscle. Fibrillations are often thought of as EMG evidence of anterior horn cell disease, but they occur with myopathy and are presumed to develop because the inflammatory muscle disease damages the connection between the neuromuscular junction and much of the motor unit. Fibrillations appear with myopathy because of denervation, but the denervation results from injury postsynaptically rather than presynaptically.

372. The answer is B. *(Lechtenberg, Synopsis, p 97.)* Myasthenia gravis is a disease, or more accurately a collection of diseases, in which autoimmune damage occurs at the neuromuscular junction. It is the postsynaptic membrane that is damaged in myasthenia gravis and it is the acetylcholine receptor that is the principal site of damage. A relative acetylcholine deficiency develops at the synapse because receptors are blocked or inefficient. Symptoms of myasthenia gravis range from slight ocular motor weakness to ventilatory failure.

373. The answer is C. *(Lechtenberg, Synopsis, pp 97–99.)* More than 90 percent of patients with myasthenia gravis have some type of ocular motor weakness. This ranges from ophthalmoplegia to lid ptosis. Patients usually notice the lid weakness or complain of blurred vision as one of the first symptoms of myasthenia. More severe disease will include limb weakness, difficulty with swallowing, and respiratory difficulties. Patients usually report fatigue that increases as the day progresses.

374. The answer is C. *(Lechtenberg, Synopsis, p 99.)* Sarcoidosis is a poorly understood inflammatory disease that may cause neuropathy as well as myopathy. Multiple organs are usually involved with sarcoidosis, with hepatic or pulmonary disease often the most consistent finding. The noncaseating granulomas help to distinguish sarcoidosis from tuberculosis, a similar disease with an established infectious basis that usually produces caseating granulomas.

375. The answer is B. *(Lechtenberg, Synopsis, p 99.)* The term *heliotrope* derives from the color of the periorbital rash characteristic of dermatomyositis. The rash is violet like parts of the sunflower called *heliotrope*. This rash surrounds both eyes and is usually associated with an erythematous rash across the knuckles. Men with dermatomyositis are at higher-than-normal risk of having underlying malignancies.

376. The answer is E. *(Lechtenberg, Synopsis, p 99.)* The causes of myopathy are remarkably diverse. Viruses, parasites, vasculitis, and endocrine disturbances may all produce myopathies with similar symptoms. Indeed, with thyroid disease, either an overactive gland or an underactive gland may be associated with a severe myopathy producing weakness. Enzymatic defects and rheumatologic diseases may produce myopathies, and in many cases the pattern of pain and weakness is remarkably similar for distinctly different diseases.

377. The answer is D. *(Johnson, ed 3. pp 400–401.)* Duchenne dystrophy has been incontrovertibly linked to the gene that makes dystrophin. The more profound the disturbance of this gene, the earlier the disease becomes symptomatic. The gene for dystrophin has single or multiple deletions in affected children. Women who are probable carriers of the defective gene can be checked for heterozygosity and given genetic counseling. Chorionic villus biopsy at 8 to 9 weeks can determine if a fetus at risk for the deletion actually carries it.

378. The answer is B. *(Johnson, ed 3. pp 399–401. Lechtenberg, Synopsis, p 94.)* Duchenne muscular dystrophy is a fairly common cause of childhood disability, but it is limited to boys. The disease is progressive, but the progression is over the course of years rather than weeks. Affected children rarely survive past adolescence. The incidence of the defect in male fetuses is greater than that in male infants because affected male fetuses have a higher rate of spontaneous abortion than do unaffected male fetuses in families carrying the abnormal gene.

379. The answer is A. *(Rowland, ed 8. p 710.)* Duchenne dystrophy may occur in the person with Turner syndrome if the inherited X chromosome carries the defective dystrophin gene. In the absence of a normal X chromosome, only the defective dystrophin will be produced. The person with Turner syndrome has only one X chromosome but is phenotypically female. Duchenne dystrophy may occur in girls with two X chromosomes if translocations of material from the normal X chromosome inactivate or eliminate the normal dystrophin gene.

380. The answer is D. *(Rowland, ed 8. pp 710–711.)* The calves are usually enlarged in the child with Duchenne dystrophy. Other clinical characteristics include a lordotic posture as weakness evolves in the hip girdle musculature. The gait becomes waddling before the child is unable to walk at all. Affected children invariably exhibit Gower's sign at some time in the evolution of their weakness. The child gets up from the floor by using his hands to walk up his legs and trunk to achieve an upright posture.

381. The answer is A. *(Rowland, ed 8. p 710.)* Despite the drain from the population of males carrying the abnormal gene, the incidence of Duchenne dystrophy is stable. Males often die before they reach sexual maturity and are too impaired after adolescence to mate. There are no changes in the ovaries of women bearing a child with Duchenne dystrophy to suggest that the mutation is arising de novo in the ovary. Women with apparently normal dystrophin genes do, however, give birth to affected sons.

382. The answer is B. *(Rowland, ed 8. p 711.)* Although profound mental retardation is not typical with Duchenne dystrophy, children with the disease characteristically perform more poorly than their siblings on objective cognitive tests. Persons with Becker's variant, the much milder form of the dystrophy that usually becomes symptomatic during adult life, may have no perceptible cognitive impairments. Women carrying the gene have normal cognitive abilities.

383. The answer is D. *(Rowland, ed 8. p 711.)* A high creatine kinase (CK) in a woman with male relatives affected by Duchenne dystrophy indicates a high probability that she is a carrier of the abnormal dystrophin gene. A normal CK, however, does not rule out the possibility that the woman is a carrier of Duchenne dystrophy. Even when a person is asymptomatic as a carrier of the gene, abnormalities in limb girdle muscles may be evident on biopsy.

384. The answer is E. *(Rowland, ed 8. p 712.)* The abnormal protein dystrophin, which appears in persons with Duchenne dystrophy, is associated with the sarcolemma. It is on the inner aspect of this membrane. Disturbances in dystrophin production probably affect the integrity of the muscle membrane. Ragged red fibers are not evident on muscle biopsy specimens from patients with Duchenne dystrophy but are seen in biopsies from persons with mitochondrial defects as the basis for myopathy.

385. The answer is A. *(Johnson, ed 3. pp 400–402.)* Men with myotonic dystrophy characteristically exhibit problems with relaxing their grip, hypersomnolence, premature baldness, testicular atrophy, and cataracts. The EMG pattern displayed by these patients is often referred to as the dive-bomber pattern because of the characteristic sound produced when the evoked action potentials are listened to. The cardiac defect that evolves in these persons usually requires pacemaker implantation to avoid sudden death. Psychiatric problems also develop in many patients with myotonic dystrophy, but their basis is unknown.

Toxic Injuries

DIRECTIONS: Each question below contains five suggested responses. Select the **one best** response to each question.

386. Parkinsonism may be produced by poisoning with any of the following agents EXCEPT

(A) lead
(B) manganese
(C) mercury
(D) carbon monoxide
(E) carbon disulfide

387. All the following medications may induce delirium EXCEPT

(A) atropine
(B) barbiturates
(C) glutethimide (Doriden)
(D) penicillin
(E) phencyclidine hydrochloride (PCP)

388. Delirium tremens is distinct from other forms of delirium in that it

(A) is intractable
(B) involves paranoid delusions
(C) is precipitated by ethanol withdrawal
(D) is a medical emergency
(E) is the effect of a primary brain disorder

389. The most common site of CNS atrophy associated with chronic alcoholism is

(A) the superior vermis
(B) Wernicke's area
(C) the supraorbital gyrus
(D) the angular gyrus
(E) the flocculus

390. The children of women exposed to methyl mercury may exhibit all the following EXCEPT

(A) microcephaly
(B) abnormal gyrations
(C) holoprosencephaly
(D) disturbances of cortical lamination
(E) heterotopic neurons in the cerebellum

391. All the following toxins routinely produce brain damage with prominent loss of cerebellar neurons EXCEPT

(A) ethanol
(B) polyvinyl chloride
(C) toluene
(D) trichloroethylene
(E) ethylene glycol

392. Thallium poisoning often produces all the following neurologic effects EXCEPT

(A) choreoathetosis
(B) seizures
(C) parkinsonism
(D) tremors
(E) dysesthesias

393. With severe lead poisoning, very young children may die of brain herniation secondary to

(A) subdural hematomas
(B) epidural hematomas
(C) intracerebral hemorrhage
(D) obstructive hydrocephalus
(E) massive brain edema

Toxic Injuries
Answers

386. The answer is A. *(Davis, p 802.)* Poisons may cause extensive basal ganglia damage and may produce parkinsonism, but they do not produce the Lewy body inclusions seen in classic Parkinson disease. MPTP, a meperidine analogue, comes closest to producing a CNS lesion similar to that observed in Parkinson disease, but histopathologic differences can be found. That a chemical can produce an irreversible Parkinson-like condition increases the likelihood that Parkinson disease occurs as a consequence of an environmental toxin. Manganese miners have long been recognized as at risk for parkinsonism as a consequence of exposure to this metal. Carbon monoxide, mercury, and carbon disulfide may also produce parkinsonism, but the symptoms associated with these poisons are more variable and less limited to the CNS than those associated with manganese poisoning.

387. The answer is D. *(Rowland, ed 8. p 3.)* Delirium is characterized by problems with attention, alterations of consciousness, impaired reaction to the environment, restlessness, and incoherence. Delusions or hallucinations may occur as part of the disturbed mental state. In many instances this thought disorder is secondary to a correctible or reversible problem, such as exposure to a drug that interferes with cognition. Hypnotics, such as barbiturates and phencyclidine; stimulants, such as amphetamines; and atropinics, such as scopolamine, are especially likely to induce delirium in susceptible persons.

388. The answer is C. *(Rowland, ed 8. p 3.)* Delirium tremens may be intractable and fatal if it is not treated, but other types of delirium are equally ominous. This type of delirium is, however, distinctly associated with chronic alcoholism. It usually develops within 2 days of ethanol withdrawal and involves tachycardia, fever, agitation, and disorientation. Treatment generally involves chlordiazepoxide (Librium) or barbiturates.

389. The answer is A. *(Davis, pp 377–388.)* The superior vermis of the cerebellum loses Purkinje cells and exhibits atrophy of the molecular layer in alcoholic persons after years or decades of ethanol use. Alcoholic patients may have gait instability and limb ataxia associated with this injury, but the clinical signs are usually fairly mild considering the histologic damage done by ethanol. White matter in the cerebellum is relatively unaffected.

390. The answer is C. *(Davis, p 183.)* Many of the defects seen in children born to women who have had excessive exposure to the neurotoxin methyl mercury involve defects in migration of neurons or of both glia and neurons. Holoprosencephaly is a defect in the division of the anterior elements of the brain. It occasionally develops in fetuses born to diabetic mothers, but it is a rare developmental defect and is not typically seen as a consequence of methyl mercury exposure. Survival with holoprosencephaly is negligible if indeed the fetus reaches maturity at all.

391. The answer is E. *(Gilman, Disorders, pp 322–326.)* Ethanol is certainly the most common cause of toxic damage to the cerebellum, simply because alcoholism is so common throughout the industrialized world. The cerebellar vermis is especially susceptible to damage from chronic ethanol excess. Alcoholic persons routinely exhibit atrophy with loss of Purkinje cells and other neural elements from the superior vermis. Antiepileptics may also produce neuronal loss, which is most prominent in the cerebellum. This has been most often observed with protracted phenytoin use. Polyvinyl chloride, toluene, and trichloroethylene may damage several different populations of cells in the cerebellum.

392. The answer is C. *(Gilman, Disorders, pp 322–323.)* Poisoning with the metal thallium may occur through industrial exposure or accidental ingestion. It is contained in some rat poisons. It affects both the central and peripheral nervous systems. Ataxia, tremors, cranial nerve palsies, seizures, and painful dysesthesias may develop with acute or chronic poisoning. Systemic evidence of thallium poisoning includes hair loss, gastrointestinal distress, and tachycardia. Parkinsonism does not develop with exposure to this poison, but other movement disorders, such as choreoathetosis, do.

393. The answer is E. *(Gilman, Disorders, p 323.)* Lead poisoning may cause ataxia and tremor in children exposed to relatively low levels. Chronic exposure routinely impairs psychomotor development and may lead to substantial retardation in very young children. Brain edema develops with toxic lead exposure in infancy and may be lethal even with efforts to relieve the intracranial pressure. Children are exposed to lead in many forms in the environment, including lead-based paint chips from old construction and lead-tainted soil in areas with heavy vehicular traffic.

Eye Disease and Visual Disturbances

DIRECTIONS: Each question below contains five suggested responses. Select the **one best** response to each question.

394. Tubular or tunnel vision in which the patient reports the same size area of perception regardless of how far from the testing screen the examination is performed often indicates

(A) retinitis pigmentosa
(B) neurosyphilis
(C) sarcoidosis
(D) chorioretinitis
(E) hysteria

395. Scotomas may develop with any of the following EXCEPT

(A) quinine ingestion
(B) ischemic optic neuropathy
(C) cataract formation
(D) tobacco-alcohol amblyopia
(E) Leber hereditary optic atrophy

396. If a homonymous hemianopia is incongruent—that is dissimilar for each eye—the lesion responsible will usually be in the

(A) optic chiasm
(B) parietal lobe
(C) occipital lobe
(D) retina
(E) optic nerve

397. Chorioretinitis may develop with any of the following EXCEPT

(A) temporal arteritis
(B) sarcoidosis
(C) toxoplasmosis
(D) tuberculosis
(E) histoplasmosis

398. The most common form of retinal degeneration is

(A) serous retinitis
(B) retinitis pigmentosa
(C) confluent drusen
(D) drug-induced retinopathy
(E) paraneoplastic retinal degeneration

399. Absence of the red reflex on ophthalmologic evaluation of the newborn probably indicates

(A) congenital cataracts
(B) chorioretinitis
(C) retinitis pigmentosa
(D) optic atrophy
(E) holoprosencephaly

400. Glaucoma develops in nearly one-third of children with

(A) neurofibromatosis type 1
(B) neurofibromatosis type 2
(C) Sturge-Weber syndrome (encephalotrigeminal angiomatosis)
(D) tuberous sclerosis
(E) Arnold-Chiari malformation

401. Retinitis caused by cytomegalovirus appears to respond to antiviral treatment with

(A) cytarabine
(B) vidarabine
(C) ribavirin
(D) interferon
(E) ganciclovir

402. The acute appearance of a large central scotoma may be precipitated by

(A) pseudotumor cerebri
(B) chronic ethanolism
(C) chlorpromazine ingestion
(D) methyl alcohol intoxication
(E) isoniazid use

403. Papillitis is easily distinguished from the papilledema of increased intracranial pressure by the

(A) degree of swelling of the optic disc
(B) homonymous hemianopia associated with it
(C) visual loss characteristic of it
(D) limitation of eye movement associated with it
(E) loss of the red reflex

Questions 404–405

A 19-year-old woman with complaints of headaches and visual blurring had prominent bulging of both optic nerve heads with obscuration of all margins of both optic discs. Her physician was reluctant to pursue neurologic studies because the patient was 8 months pregnant and had had similar complaints during the last month of another pregnancy. Her physical and neurologic examination was otherwise unrevealing.

404. If neuroimaging studies had been performed on this woman, they probably would have revealed

(A) a subfrontal meningioma
(B) intraventricular blood
(C) slitlike ventricles
(D) transtentorial herniation
(E) metastatic breast carcinoma

405. The treatment of choice for this young woman is

(A) lumbar puncture
(B) cesarean section
(C) induction of labor
(D) vitamin A supplements
(E) acetazolamide

406. A young man with multiple sclerosis exhibited paradoxical dilation of the right pupil when a flashlight was redirected from the left eye into the right eye. Swinging the flashlight back to the left eye produced constriction of the right pupil. This patient apparently has

(A) early cataract formation in the right eye
(B) occipital lobe damage on the left
(C) oscillopsia
(D) hippus
(E) optic atrophy

407. A 23-year-old woman complained of 2 days of visual loss associated with discomfort in the right eye. She appeared otherwise healthy, but her family reported recurrent problems with bladder control over the prior 2 years, which the patient was reluctant to discuss. On neurologic examination, this young woman exhibited dysmetria in her right arm, a plantar extensor response of the left foot, and slurred speech. The most informative ancillary test would be expected to be

(A) visual evoked response testing
(B) sural nerve biopsy
(C) electroencephalography
(D) MR scanning
(E) CT scanning

408. All the following will produce optic atrophy EXCEPT

(A) traumatic transection of the optic nerve
(B) retinal hemangioblastoma
(C) neurosyphilis
(D) multiple sclerosis
(E) optic nerve glioma

409. Injuries to the macula or fovea centralis may produce a loss in acuity of as much as

(A) 10 percent
(B) 20 percent
(C) 40 percent
(D) 75 percent
(E) 95 percent

410. The most obvious changes in the retina with chronic hypertension routinely include

(A) retinal tears
(B) optic atrophy
(C) segmental narrowing of arterioles
(D) drusen
(E) telangiectasias

411. Retinal microaneurysms most often occur with

(A) sarcoidosis
(B) chronic hypertension
(C) diabetes mellitus
(D) anterior communicating aneurysms
(E) chorioretinitis

412. The ocular motor nerve most likely to be impaired if the patient acutely develops diplopia is

(A) oculomotor
(B) trochlear
(C) abducens
(D) ciliary
(E) Müller's

413. A child acutely developing a sixth nerve (abducens) palsy is at most risk for a

(A) pontine glioma
(B) medullary glioma
(C) mesencephalic infarction
(D) pontine infarction
(E) medullary infarction

414. Facial pain and diplopia (Gradenigo syndrome) in a child is usually caused by

(A) ischemia
(B) infection
(C) neoplasm
(D) trauma
(E) hemorrhage

415. The ocular motor muscle most likely to be injured with facial trauma is that innervated by the

(A) superior division of the third cranial nerve
(B) inferior division of the third cranial nerve
(C) fourth (trochlear) cranial nerve
(D) sixth (abducens) cranial nerve
(E) long ciliary nerve

416. Varicella-zoster ophthalmicus most commonly affects which ocular motor nerve?

(A) Superior division of the third
(B) Inferior division of the third
(C) Fourth (trochlear)
(D) Sixth (abducens)
(E) Long ciliary

417. The initial sign of pressure on the third nerve is usually impaired

(A) adduction
(B) abduction
(C) depression
(D) elevation
(E) pupillary contraction

418. A third nerve palsy associated with diabetes mellitus is usually characterized by

(A) poor pupillodilation
(B) poor pupilloconstriction
(C) sparing of pupillary function
(D) inversion of the affected eye
(E) upward deviation of the affected eye

419. Pupillary constriction occurring with attempted adduction of the globe suggests

(A) mesencephalic infarction
(B) pontine glioma
(C) acute glaucoma
(D) iridocyclitis
(E) aberrant third nerve regeneration

420. Acute bilateral ophthalmoplegia suggests each of the following
EXCEPT

(A) pretectal infarction
(B) posterior communicating artery
aneurysm
(C) Wernicke disease
(D) tuberculous meningitis
(E) myasthenia gravis

421. Evidence of the medial longitudinal fasciculus (MLF) syndrome invariably means

(A) a mesencephalic or pontine in-
jury
(B) a brainstem glioma
(C) multiple sclerosis
(D) diabetes mellitus
(E) basilar artery aneurysm

422. The most likely diagnosis in a
30-year-old woman with evidence of
bilateral injury to the medial longitudinal fasciculus (MLF) is

(A) progressive supranuclear palsy
(B) multiple sclerosis
(C) subacute sclerosing panencepha-
litis
(D) progressive multifocal leuko-
encephalopathy
(E) botulism

423. The most common cause of induced nystagmus is

(A) hysteria
(B) drug intoxication
(C) eye strain
(D) myopia
(E) hypermetropia

424. The child with rapid downward
deviation of both eyes followed by
slow upward conjugate eye movements probably has

(A) subacute sclerosing
panencephalitis
(B) multiple sclerosis
(C) pontine glioma
(D) cervicomedullary junction
ischemia
(E) cerebral palsy

425. Rhythmical jerk nystagmus elicited by having the patient look at a
rotating drum with stripes on it suggests

(A) drug toxicity
(B) brainstem ischemia
(C) Parinaud syndrome
(D) unilateral parietal lobe damage
(E) no pathologic lesion in the brain

426. A 36-year-old man abruptly
loses vision in one eye. His retina appears cloudy and grayish yellow with
narrowed arterioles. The fovea appears cherry red and the vessels that
are obvious appear to have seg-
mented columns of blood. This man
probably has

(A) chorioretinitis
(B) occlusion of the central retinal
vein
(C) occlusion of the central retinal
artery
(D) optic neuritis
(E) Tay-Sachs disease

427. Pain in or about the eye or more diffuse headache is routinely produced by all the following ocular problems EXCEPT

(A) iridocyclitis
(B) medial longitudinal fasciculus (MLF) syndrome
(C) acute glaucoma
(D) hypermetropia
(E) astigmatism

428. An acute neuro-ophthalmologic problem requiring immediate attention is often signified by each of the following EXCEPT

(A) anterior chamber hemorrhage
(B) monocular ophthalmoplegia
(C) acute amaurosis
(D) subconjunctival hemorrhage
(E) persistent pupillary dilatation

429. Amaurosis fugax usually arises because of disease in the

(A) middle cerebral artery
(B) posterior cerebral artery
(C) anterior cerebral artery
(D) internal carotid artery
(E) anterior choroidal artery

430. Horner syndrome includes all the following elements EXCEPT

(A) ptosis
(B) miosis
(C) mydriasis
(D) anhidrosis
(E) unequal pupils

431. A 5-year-old girl cut her face on broken glass. Initially the injury appeared superficial except for a small area of deeper penetration just above the right eyebrow. Within 4 days, the child complained of periorbital pain and double vision. The tissues about the eye were erythematous and the eye appeared to bulge slightly. The optic disc was sharp and no afferent pupillary defect was apparent. Visual acuity in the affected eye was preserved. This child probably has

(A) orbital cellulitis
(B) cavernous sinus thrombosis
(C) transverse sinus thrombosis
(D) optic neuritis
(E) diphtheritic polyneuropathy

432. An otherwise healthy young woman has poorly responsive pupils that are tonically dilated. A careful neurologic examination reveals bilaterally absent Achilles tendon jerks. This woman probably has

(A) a cervical spinal cord tumor
(B) a brainstem glioma
(C) multiple sclerosis
(D) peripheral neuropathy
(E) benign pupillary dilatation

433. With neurosyphilis, the pupil is likely to be

(A) completely normal
(B) small and irregular in shape
(C) dilated and irregular in shape
(D) small and regular in shape
(E) dilated and regular in shape

DIRECTIONS: The group of questions below consists of lettered representations followed by a set of numbered items. For each numbered item select the **one** lettered representation with which it is **most** closely associated. Each lettered representation may be used **once, more than once, or not at all.**

Questions 434–438

For each clinical scenario, select the probable visual field discovered on tangent screen testing as depicted below.

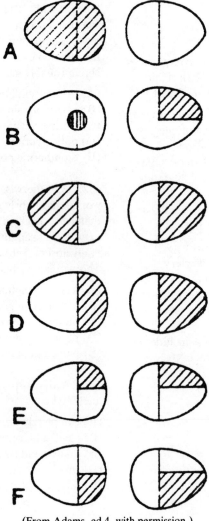

(From Adams, ed 4, with permission.)

434. A 30-year-old woman with diabetes mellitus and menstrual irregularities complained of chronic headaches with blurring of vision. On examination she had a lantern jaw, prominent nose, spade-shaped hands, and prominent supraorbital ridges. She was slightly taller than other members of her family

435. A 17-year-old woman with recurrent enuresis noticed pain and visual problems in her left eye. She had had transient weakness in both legs for 2 days 6 months prior to the development of the visual difficulty. Her parents had noted slurring and slowing of her speech that appeared to persist long after the transient gait ataxia and leg weakness had resolved

436. A 40-year-old man suffered a gunshot wound to the back of the head. An MR scan revealed extensive damage to the left occipital lobe with sparing of the right occipital lobe

437. A 51-year-old woman complained of progressive loss of visual acuity in her left eye. Over the course of 5 years her acuity had deteriorated from 20/20 to 20/400. An MR of her brain revealed a large meningioma impinging on the left side of the optic chiasm. There was no associated hydrocephalus

438. A 65-year-old man developed language problems with no loss of consciousness. He was found to have a receptive aphasia and an MR scan confirmed an area of infarction in the left temporal lobe confined to structures above and lateral to the temporal horn of the lateral ventricle

Eye Disease and Visual Disturbances

Answers

394. The answer is E. *(Adams, ed 4. p 201.)* Tunnel vision must be distinguished from concentric constriction. In the latter the area perceived enlarges as the test screen is moved farther away from the patient, but the overall visual field is always smaller than the normal visual field. Concentric constriction associated with optic atrophy may develop with neurosyphilis. Tunnel vision is not a physiologic pattern of visual loss. Patients with true visual loss may, however, elaborate on their visual loss and report such improbable field patterns or exhibit a shrinking visual field as the examination continues. This spiraling of the visual field reflects stress or panic and should not be construed as evidence of a normal visual field.

395. The answer is C. *(Adams, ed 4. pp 202–203.)* A scotoma is an area of visual loss surrounded by areas of normal vision. It is usually used in the context of retinal or optic nerve damage, rather than in reference to optic chiasm, optic tract, lateral geniculate, optic radiation, or occipital lobe disease. Damage to these components of the visual system behind the optic nerves usually produces visual field defects that extend to the edges of the visual field at least at one point. A physiologic blind spot exists because there are no photoreceptors at the point on the retina where the optic nerve exits the eye.

396. The answer is B. *(Adams, ed 4. pp 202–203.)* To have a homonymous hemianopia, the patient must have a lesion in the visual pathway behind the optic chiasm. Lesions in the occipital lobe usually produce highly congruous field cuts. The more anterior in the optic radiation coursing through the temporal and parietal lobes the lesion is, the more incongruous the hemianopic field cuts will be.

397. The answer is A. *(Adams, ed 4. p 198.)* In chorioretinitis both the choroidal membrane supporting the retina and the retina itself are damaged.

Damage to the pigment epithelium of the choroid produces a punched-out appearance to the lesions. Collections of dark pigment are juxtaposed on backgrounds of bright yellow. Congenital chorioretinitis occurs with several different infectious agents, including toxoplasma, cytomegalovirus, and syphilis.

398. The answer is B. *(Adams, ed 4. pp 198–199.)* Retinitis pigmentosa is a hereditary degenerative disease involving the retinal receptors and adjacent pigment cells. As this degeneration progresses, small accumulations of pigment appear about the periphery of the retina. Optic disc pallor is evident later in the disease. Retinitis pigmentosa develops along with Bassen-Kornzweig disease (abetalipoproteinemia), Refsum disease, and other metabolic disorders producing extensive nervous system damage.

399. The answer is A. *(Adams, ed 4. pp 190–192.)* On shining a light through the pupil of the normal newborn, the normal color of the retina is perceived as an orange-red reflection of the light. Failure to perceive that reflection usually indicates opacification of the pathway of light transmission. Several types of intrauterine infections, including rubella and cytomegalovirus infection, may produce congenital cataracts.

400. The answer is C. *(Rowland, ed 8. pp 582–583.)* Children with this disorder have large port-wine spots on their faces, contralateral hemiparesis, retardation, and seizures, as well as glaucoma. Skull radiographs reveal intracranial calcifications that are associated with leptomeningeal angiomatosis. This syndrome results from a defect on chromosome 3.

401. The answer is E. *(Johnson, ed 3. p 112.)* All the drugs listed have antiviral activity with effects on CMV in vitro. Ganciclovir is the only one with demonstrable clinical effects on CMV infection. This drug is a 2-deoxyguanosine analogue and has been used for CMV pneumonia and gastroenteritis, as well as chorioretinitis.

402. The answer is D. *(Adams, ed 4. pp 200–201.)* Persons who ingest methyl alcohol will usually be very ill if they survive. Acidosis is a life-threatening complication of exposure to this toxin. Isoniazid, ethambutol, streptomycin, and other drugs may produce similar field cuts, but the blind spots developing with these toxins usually appear subacutely or chronically rather than abruptly.

403. The answer is C. *(Adams, ed 4. p 200.)* Visual loss is usually substantial with papillitis, an inflammation of the optic nerve head, and inconsequential with papilledema. Patients with papillitis usually also complain of pain on moving the globe and sensitivity to light pressure on the globe. About one out of ten patients will have both eyes involved simultaneously. Papillitis is often an early sign of multiple sclerosis.

404. The answer is C. *(Lechtenberg, Synopsis, p 112.)* Although papilledema must be considered evidence of a potentially life-threatening intracranial process, optic nerve bulging in this young woman is most likely from pseudotumor cerebri. This is a relatively benign condition that occasionally develops in obese or pregnant women. CSF pressure is markedly elevated in these patients, but they are not at risk of herniation. The condition is presumed to arise from hormonal problems. Without treatment, the increased intracranial pressure will produce optic nerve damage with loss of visual acuity.

405. The answer is A. *(Lechtenberg, Synopsis, pp 112–113.)* With pseudotumor cerebri, removal of some of the CSF produces a protracted lowering of the intracranial pressure. This pressure reduction is desirable because persistent pressure elevations will damage the optic nerve. Pseudotumor cerebri in the pregnant woman usually abates soon after the fetus leaves its mother, but this condition is not serious enough to justify termination or acceleration of a pregnancy. Vitamin excess may cause pseudotumor in some persons. Diuretics are sometimes used to manage patients who are not pregnant, but they are usually less effective than repeated lumbar puncture when that is practical.

406. The answer is E. *(Lechtenberg, Synopsis, pp 57–58.)* The test performed is usually called the *swinging flashlight test,* and the pupillary finding is a Marcus Gunn or afferent pupillary defect. It commonly develops in persons with multiple sclerosis as a sequela of optic neuritis. Damage to the optic nerve reduces the light perceived with the affected eye. If the other eye has less or no optic atrophy, the consensual response of the pupil to light perceived by the better eye will constrict the pupil in the atrophic eye, even though direct light to the injured eye does not elicit a strong pupillary constriction.

407. The answer is D. *(Lechtenberg, Multiple Sclerosis, pp 69–81.)* This young woman almost certainly has multiple sclerosis. Her visual loss can be explained by optic neuritis. Her bladder problems may be from demyelination of corticospinal tract fibers. Many patients are reluctant to discuss minor problems with bladder, bowel, or sexual function with a physician of the opposite sex. The positive Babinski sign, focal dysmetria, and apparent dysarthria all support the diagnosis of a multifocal central nervous system lesion. Multiple lesions disseminated in time and space are typical of multiple sclerosis. With MR scanning, the multifocal areas of demyelination should be apparent. Many more lesions may be evident on MR scanning than are suggested by the physical examination.

408. The answer is B. *(Adams, ed 4. p 202.)* With optic atrophy the nerve may become chalky white and have a distinctly demarcated margin. A similar appearance may develop in persons with severe myopia (nearsightedness). Retinal hemangioblastomas may produce a substantial loss of vision, but the optic disc will still appear normal.

409. The answer is E. *(Adams, ed 4. pp 194–195.)* The cones of the retina are packed into the macula, and the primary focus of the lens is at the macula. The macula is usually evident on ophthalmologic examination because it normally reflects a point of light that can be seen through the ophthalmoscope. It is located 3 to 4 mm temporally from the optic disc.

410. The answer is C. *(Adams, ed 4. pp 195–196.)* The vessels apparent on funduscopic examination of the retina are arterioles and venules. In addition to segmental narrowing of arterioles, the retina may exhibit arteriolar straightening and arteriolar-venular compression. The thickened arteriolar wall compresses the venule at the point it crosses it, a pattern often referred to as nicking.

411. The answer is C. *(Adams, ed 4. p 197.)* These aneurysms appear as small, red dots on the surface of the retina. They may appear as one of the first manifestations of diabetes mellitus and are rarely larger than 90 microns across. They may be more obvious in green light. A proliferative retinopathy may occur along with these microaneurysms in the patient with diabetes mellitus.

412. The answer is C. *(Adams, ed 4. p 215.)* Injury to the sixth nerve produces a lateral rectus palsy. This type of ocular motor paresis is twice as common as a third nerve palsy and six times as common as fourth nerve problems. With lateral rectus weakness the affected eye will remain inverted on attempts to look straight ahead.

413. The answer is A. *(Adams, ed 4. p 215.)* An abducens dysfunction with lateral rectus palsy may develop in children with increased intracranial pressure or with direct damage to the brainstem. With a brainstem glioma, both brainstem damage and increased intracranial pressure may develop secondary to the tumor. The adult developing an acute abducens palsy is also at high risk for tumor. Metastatic lesions from the nasopharynx are especially likely in the adult, but vascular disease is also a significant cause of ocular motor dysfunction in adults, especially in the elderly.

414. The answer is B. *(Adams, ed 4. p 215.)* Gradenigo syndrome arises with an osteomyelitis of the petrous pyramid. The abducens and trigeminal nerves are affected as they pass close to the tip of the petrous bone. Chronic ear infections may extend to the petrous pyramid and produce this syndrome if they are not properly managed.

415. The answer is C. *(Adams, ed 4. p 215.)* The fourth cranial nerve innervates the superior oblique muscle. Because this muscle extends far anterior in the orbit, it is at high risk of injury with trauma to the orbit or the full face. The third nerve is especially vulnerable to pressure from aneurysms, but it is usually not disturbed with head trauma unless there are local fractures impinging upon it. Injury to the fourth nerve with facial trauma will usually induce a slight head tilt. The head tilt compensates for impaired intorsion of the affected eye.

416. The answer is C. *(Adams, ed 4. pp 215–216.)* Varicella zoster, previously known as "herpes zoster," spreads to the face along the trigeminal nerve. The fourth nerve is presumably involved because it shares its nerve sheath with the ophthalmic division of the trigeminal nerve. The third and sixth nerves may also be involved with varicella zoster, but this occurs much less frequently than involvement of the fourth nerve.

417. The answer is E. *(Adams, ed 4. p 216.)* The pupilloconstrictor fibers of the third nerve lie superficially on the nerve. Lesions compressing the nerve impinge upon these fibers before they disturb the ocular motor fibers. The third nerve is not involved in abduction of the globe; this is accomplished by the abducens nerve, which controls the lateral rectus muscle.

418. The answer is C. *(Adams, ed 4. p 216.)* The vessel usually obstructed with diabetic third nerve injury is deep in the third nerve. The superficial fibers to the iris are supplied by a separate set of vessels, and these are usually spared with diabetes mellitus. The affected person may complain of pain in and about the eye with the damaged third nerve.

419. The answer is E. *(Adams, ed 4. p 216.)* Oculomotor fibers that have been damaged reversibly may regenerate and connect to the wrong target. This aberrant regeneration is seen most often with lesions that chronically compress the third nerve. Aneurysms, cholesteatomas, and neoplasms should be suspected in the person exhibiting this type of disturbance.

420. The answer is B. *(Adams, ed 4. p 216.)* A posterior communicating aneurysm may produce ophthalmoplegia by compressing a third nerve, but bilateral injury does not occur. Other considerations in the patient with acutely evolving ocular motor dysfunction include the Miller-Fisher variant of the Guillain-Barré syndrome and botulism. Lesions affecting both cavernous sinuses simultaneously do occur and must be sought when bilateral ophthalmoplegia occurs.

421. The answer is A. *(Adams, ed 4. pp 216–217.)* In the MLF syndrome, the patient has incomplete adduction ipsilateral to the lesion in the MLF on conjugate lateral gaze. On attempted conjugate lateral gaze away from the side of the lesion, the patient has nystagmus in the abducting eye. The fast component of the nystagmus is directed temporally.

422. The answer is B. *(Adams, ed 4. pp 216–217.)* Vascular disease may produce bilateral injury to the MLF in the elderly, but it is an unlikely explanation in the young adult. Injury to the MLF in multiple sclerosis is demyelinating. Bilateral MLF syndromes associated with optic atrophy are virtually diagnostic of multiple sclerosis in persons under 40 years of age.

423. The answer is B. *(Adams, ed 4. p 218.)* Alcohol and barbiturates are the drugs that most often cause nystagmus. A variety of hypnotic and antiepileptic drugs are also often implicated because they are widely used by the general population. Although the severity of nystagmus in the two eyes may be unequal, the severity is invariably worse in the horizontal plane of gaze when the nystagmus is an adverse effect of drug use.

424. The answer is C. *(Adams, ed 4. p 219.)* The phenomenon described is commonly referred to as *ocular bobbing*. It is an involuntary movement that usually develops with pontine damage. Damage to the cerebellum occasionally produces a similar disturbance of eye movements.

425. The answer is E. *(Adams, ed 4. p 219.)* This type of nystagmus is called *optokinetic nystagmus*. It is a pattern of eye movements that should be elicitable with the normal patient. If the nystagmus is less obvious on rotating the drum in one direction, the patient may have a parietal lesion responsible for the asymmetric response.

426. The answer is C. *(Adams, ed 4. p 197.)* Occlusion of the central retinal artery may be from atheromatous particles, fibrin-platelet emboli, or local retinal artery compression. The visual loss is usually painless and irreversible. Occlusion of the internal carotid artery, the artery from which the ophthalmic and ultimately the retinal arteries originate, need not produce ischemic damage to the retina if collateral supply to the retinal artery is sufficient.

427. The answer is B. *(Adams, ed 4. p 137.)* Hypermetropia (farsightedness) and astigmatism produce headache because the victims of these refractive problems involuntarily try to correct for the poor focus achieved by chronically contracting extraocular, frontal, temporal, and occipital muscles. With acute glaucoma the raised intraocular pressure usually produces pain in the affected eye that radiates to the forehead. Any inflammatory lesion of the eye, such as iridocyclitis, may cause considerable pain in the eye.

428. The answer is D. *(Adams, ed 4. p 208. Lechtenberg, Multiple Sclerosis, pp 41–42; Synopsis, p 118.)* Subconjunctival hemorrhage is likely to be from local trauma but does occasionally develop as an early sign of a coagulation defect or even as a persistent manifestation of seizure activity. The trauma responsible for the hemorrhage is usually inconsequential and the presence of subconjunctival blood poses no threat to vision. Acute amaurosis, that is loss of vision, may be from optic neuritis, rapidly evolving glaucoma, or optic nerve ischemia and must always be investigated. Pupillary dilatation and paralysis associated with monocular amaurosis suggest a rapidly evolving glaucoma and must be managed on an emergency basis to avoid permanent visual loss. Monocular ophthalmoplegia may develop with diabetes mellitus, but in the absence of known diabetes, possible causes of this deficit include a posterior communicating artery aneurysm. Anterior chamber hemorrhage may lead to permanent loss of vision unless it is managed on an emergency basis.

429. The answer is D. *(Toole, ed 4. p 78.)* Emboli arising in or traveling through the internal carotid artery may exit to the ophthalmic artery and cause obstruction. The transient ischemia that occurs before the embolus breaks up usually produces transient visual loss in the ipsilateral eye. Amaurosis fugax is by definition a fleeting loss of vision.

430. The answer is C. *(Lechtenberg, Synopsis, p 11.)* Mydriasis indicates enlargement of the pupil, and in Horner syndrome the affected pupil is small and relatively poorly reactive to light. The injury responsible for the syndrome is in the sympathetic supply to the face. The site of injury may be in the hypothalamus, brainstem, or cervical cord or along the sympathetic nerve supply to the face.

431. The answer is A. *(Adams, ed 4. pp 213–216.)* The fact that vision is preserved excludes optic neuritis and cavernous sinus thrombosis. Optic neuritis will produce pain in the affected eye and may be associated with a normal optic disc, but visual acuity should be deficient and an afferent pupillary defect should be apparent. Cavernous sinus thrombosis usually produces proptosis and pain, but impaired venous drainage from the eye should interfere with acuity, and the retina should appear profoundly disturbed. With a diphtheritic polyneuropathy, an ophthalmoplegia may develop, but this would not be limited to one eye and is not usually associated with facial trauma. Transverse sinus thrombosis may produce cerebrocortical dysfunction or stroke, but ophthalmoplegia would not be a manifestation of this problem.

432. The answer is E. *(Lechtenberg, Synopsis, p 11.)* The pupillary abnormality is called Adie's tonic pupil. It is usually seen in young women who are otherwise healthy and may occur in isolation or in association with absent tendon reflexes. Local trauma to the eye should be considered if only one pupil is affected. If both pupils are affected, drug use should be considered. In most cases this is a totally benign phenomenon.

433. The answer is B. *(Lechtenberg, Synopsis, p 11.)* With neurosyphilis the patient may develop an Argyll Robertson pupil. The pupil is usually poorly reactive to light, small, and irregular in shape. Both eyes or only one eye may be affected. Although reactivity to light is deficient, pupillary accommodation with changes in distance from the eye is usually good. The pupillary reaction may, however, be complicated by optic atrophy, which also may develop as a consequence of neurosyphilis.

434. The answer is C. *(Adams, ed 4. pp 194–195.)* This woman has acromegaly, presumably as a result of a pituitary tumor. The growth hormone–secreting tumor responsible will compress the optic chiasm as it extends superiorly out of the sella turcica. Transsphenoidal resection of the tumor may be feasible if the tumor has not extended too far to the side of the sella turcica. Pressure on the optic chiasm will produce a bitemporal hemianopia.

435. The answer is A. *(Adams, ed 4. pp 194–195.)* Multiple sclerosis probably caused the ataxia, paraparesis, and dysarthria evident in this young woman. Her loss of vision was presumably from optic neuritis. This would typically affect only one eye at a time, but the other eye would eventually be involved by the disease. The loss of vision would be for the entire visual field of one eye acutely. As the monocular blindness cleared, the patient would be left with an enlarged blind spot.

436. The answer is D. *(Adams, ed 4. pp 194–195.)* Damage to the left calcarine cortex of the occipital lobe will produce a right homonymous hemianopia. This will usually split the field of vision exactly at its point of fixation. In rare instances, macular vision from both eyes is preserved, a phenomenon usually referred to as *macular sparing*.

437. The answer is B. *(Adams, ed 4. pp 194–195.)* With a lesion impinging upon the chiasm from one side, there should be a field cut in the contralateral field of the contralateral eye. The ipsilateral eye may exhibit little more than an enlarged blind spot that impinges upon central vision, a pattern called a *centrocecal scotoma*. With more substantial damage to the fibers from the eye ipsilateral to the chiasmatic lesion, the patient may have a left nasal hemianopia, but this rarely appears.

438. The answer is E. *(Adams, ed 4. pp 194–195.)* Temporal lobe damage produces a superior homonymous quandrantanopia if there is damage to the optic radiation from the lateral geniculate. Only the lower fibers in this radiation swing superficially in the temporal lobe, extending in front of the temporal horn of the lateral ventricle before swinging back as Meyer's loop to connections in the occipital lobe. Fibers for the superior visual field are in the lower part of the optic radiation.

Disturbances of Hearing, Balance, Smell, and Taste

DIRECTIONS: Each question below contains five suggested responses. Select the **one best** response to each question.

439. Presbycusis probably develops in most of the affected elderly because of

(A) calcification of ligaments stabilizing the ossicles
(B) weakness of the tensor tympani
(C) neuronal degeneration
(D) weakness of the stapedius muscle
(E) granulation tissue in the middle ear

440. With testing of the far-field brainstem auditory evoked response (FBAER), loss of the first positive deflection on the recording (wave I) may indicate disease in the

(A) auditory nerve
(B) cochlear nuclei in the pons
(C) superior olivary nucleus
(D) lateral lemniscus
(E) inferior colliculus of the midbrain

441. Any of the following may produce a conductive deafness EXCEPT

(A) cholesteatoma
(B) chronic otitis
(C) otosclerosis
(D) occlusion of the external auditory canal
(E) acoustic nerve schwannoma

442. Dominant temporal lobe infarction will not produce complete deafness because

(A) there is no temporal lobe representation for hearing
(B) each cochlear nucleus projects to both temporal lobes
(C) deafness results with non-dominant hemisphere damage
(D) both thalamic and temporal lobe damage must occur
(E) both brainstem and temporal lobe damage must occur

443. With disease of the middle ear, sound transmitted strictly by air conduction will be perceived as

(A) louder than that by bone conduction
(B) quieter than that by bone conduction
(C) lower-pitched than that by bone conduction
(D) higher-pitched than that by bone conduction
(E) oscillating between high and low pitch

444. With an aggressive mastoiditis, affected persons may develop a receptive aphasia as a result of extension of the infection into the

(A) frontal lobe
(B) parietal lobe
(C) temporal lobe
(D) occipital lobe
(E) cerebellum

445. Acoustic trauma from explosions, loud music, or industrial activities most commonly produces

(A) high-tone sensorineural loss
(B) low-tone sensorineural loss
(C) high-tone conductive loss
(D) low-tone conductive loss
(E) central deafness

446. All the following drugs may cause irreversible hearing loss EXCEPT

(A) streptomycin
(B) acetylsalicylic acid
(C) kanamycin
(D) neomycin
(E) gentamicin

447. Injury to any of the following might be expected to produce vertigo EXCEPT

(A) cristae of the semicircular canals
(B) spiral ganglion neurons
(C) saccular macula
(D) utricular macula
(E) the labyrinth

448. Cerebellar damage may be associated with severe vertigo if the tissue damaged is in the distribution of the

(A) superior cerebellar artery
(B) posterior inferior cerebellar artery
(C) anterior inferior cerebellar artery
(D) anterior spinal artery
(E) posterior cerebral artery

449. With vertigo developing on extreme extension or rotation of the head, the patient probably has insufficiency in the

(A) left subclavian artery
(B) internal carotid arteries bilaterally
(C) vertebrobasilar system
(D) internal maxillary artery
(E) innominate artery

450. Early in the evolution of Ménière's disease, hearing is lost

(A) over all frequencies
(B) primarily over high frequencies
(C) primarily over mid frequencies
(D) primarily over low frequencies
(E) in virtually no patients

451. Vertigo associated with a toxic labyrinthitis may appear after taking

(A) gentamicin
(B) kanamycin
(C) streptomycin
(D) acetylsalicylic acid
(E) penicillin

452. With Ménière's disease, patients are likely to complain of paroxysmal episodes of all the following EXCEPT

(A) hearing loss
(B) tinnitus
(C) amblyopia
(D) nausea
(E) vertigo

453. Tinnitus is most commonly exacerbated by

(A) alcohol
(B) aspirin
(C) glucose
(D) diazepam
(E) steroids

454. The tumor most likely to occur in persons with multiple café au lait spots is the

(A) medulloblastoma
(B) acoustic schwannoma
(C) neurofibroma
(D) ependymoma
(E) meningioma

455. Acoustic schwannomas or neuromas are most likely to develop bilaterally with

(A) type 1 neurofibromatosis (von Recklinghausen's disease)
(B) type 2 neurofibromatosis
(C) meningeal carcinomatosis
(D) multifocal meningiomas
(E) disseminated ependymomas

456. The olfactory cortex in humans is located in the

(A) anterior perforated substance
(B) lateral olfactory gyrus (prepiriform area)
(C) posterior third of the first temporal gyrus
(D) angular gyrus
(E) calcarine cortex

457. The hypogonadism and anosmia of Kallman's syndrome usually attract medical attention during

(A) the newborn period
(B) infancy
(C) childhood
(D) adolescence
(E) adult life

458. The primary modalities of taste include all the following EXCEPT

(A) sweet
(B) sour
(C) salty
(D) acidic
(E) bitter

459. Anosmia develops with head injuries because

(A) subarachnoid blood causes pial adhesions on the olfactory nerve
(B) injury to the temporal tip injures the olfactory cortex
(C) torsion on the brainstem injures trigeminal tracts
(D) shearing forces sever filaments of the receptor cells as they cross the cribriform plate
(E) traction on the chorda tympani damages fibers as they course through the skull

460. Unilateral anosmia associated with ipsilateral optic atrophy and contralateral papilledema is most likely from

(A) pseudotumor cerebri
(B) multiple sclerosis
(C) olfactory groove meningioma
(D) craniopharyngioma
(E) nasopharyngeal carcinoma

Disturbances of Hearing, Balance, Smell, and Taste

Answers

439. The answer is C. *(Adams, ed 4. p 233.)* Presbycusis is the most common cause of hearing loss in the elderly. High-frequency perception is impaired in this disorder because of sensorineural damage. The neurons most likely affected in this degenerative disorder are the spiral ganglion neurons of the cochlea.

440. The answer is A. *(Adams, ed 4. pp 28–30.)* There are seven positive waves elicited during the first 10 ms of the far-field brainstem auditory evoked response (FBAER). The stimulus used to elicit the deflections recorded is a clicking noise. The last positive deflection of the FBAER is believed to reflect the cortical response to the click stimulus.

441. The answer is E. *(Adams, ed 4. p 230.)* Conductive hearing losses are only those in which the defect is before the cochlea. Any problem interfering with transmission of sound through the external auditory canal, across the tympanic membrane, or along the ossicles of the middle ear qualifies as a basis for conductive hearing loss. Disease of the cochlea or cochlear division of the eighth cranial nerve may produce sensorineural deafness. Damage to the brainstem or brain may produce central deafness.

442. The answer is B. *(Adams, ed 4. p 230.)* Hearing in each ear is represented bilaterally even at the level of the brainstem. Lesions rarely produce sufficient damage in the brainstem to cause unilateral deafness unless they are so massive that the patient is unlikely to be responsive to most stimuli and unlikely to survive. If there is unilateral deafness, the patient should be evaluated to determine whether the hearing loss is conductive or sensorineural.

443. The answer is B. *(Adams, ed 4. p 230.)* The traditional test for detecting conductive deafness is the Rinne test. The vibrating tuning fork is applied to the mastoid process. When the patient can no longer hear the vibration of the fork, it is taken off the skull and moved to the external auditory meatus. With nerve deafness, acuity may be generally reduced, but perception with air conduction will be superior to that with bone conduction. In normal persons this will also be true. With a conductive hearing loss, the sound waves are transmitted more effectively to the cochlea directly through the bones of the skull than through the air and along the pathway that starts at the external auditory meatus.

444. The answer is C. *(Gilman, Disorders, pp 311–314.)* Mastoiditis may extend either supratentorially into the temporal lobe or infratentorially into the cerebellum. Cerebellar involvement is likely to produce ataxia, vertigo, nausea, vomiting, and morning headache. Temporal lobe extension causes a receptive aphasia by damaging Wernicke's area in the superior temporal gyrus. The lesion in either the cerebellum or the temporal lobe is usually an abscess formed by bacteria responsible for the mastoiditis. Surgical removal of the abscess is essential in either location. Progression of the abscess in either the cerebellum or the temporal lobe will be lethal.

445. The answer is A. *(Adams, ed 4. p 233.)* The principal site of damage with acoustic trauma is in the cochlea. Mechanical trauma may produce a high-tone conductive loss by perforating the eardrum. A strictly acoustic insult would not be expected to convey enough energy to the typanum to disrupt it, but it may convey enough energy to the cochlea to shear off receptor filaments from hair cells.

446. The answer is B. *(Adams, ed 4. p 233.)* Both acetylsalicylic acid (aspirin) and quinine may disturb hearing transiently, but they would not be expected to produce permanent damage. Streptomycin, neomycin, kanamycin, and gentamicin are all antimicrobial agents toxic to the ear. They cause a sensorineural hearing loss by damaging cochlear hair cells.

447. The answer is B. *(Adams, ed 4. p 237.)* The saccule, macule, and semicircular canals contain endolymph and sensory cells for the perception of changes in posture and acceleration. The spiral ganglion serves the cochlea, not the labyrinthine organ for position and rotation. The saccule and utricle have hair cells in their maculae with otoliths attached to the hairs so that gravitational effects of changes in posture may be amplified.

448. The answer is B. *(Adams, ed 4. p 240.)* The posterior inferior cerebellar artery has both medial and lateral branches. The medial branches supply the brainstem. With occlusion of these, vestibular nuclei in the brainstem are infarcted, and vertigo is common. Even with an occlusion limited to the lateral branches, vertigo is likely. If no brainstem damage occurs, cerebellar flocculonodular lobule injury may induce vertigo.

449. The answer is C. *(Adams, ed 4. p 240.)* The vertebral arteries ascend through foramina in the transverse processes of the cervical vertebrae. With bony spurs on the vertebrae or with severe atherosclerotic disease in the vertebral arteries, flow through the vertebrobasilar system may be transiently reduced when the head is extended or rotated. Because vertigo may be positional without any associated vascular insufficiency, a diagnosis of vertebrobasilar ischemia should be reached only after other causes, such as a cerebellar tumor, have been eliminated.

450. The answer is D. *(Adams, ed 4. p 241.)* Unlike the deficit of presbycusis, lower tones are those most susceptible to impaired perception during the initial phases of Ménière's disease. The severity of the hearing loss typically fluctuates considerably. As fluctuations in the low-tone loss abate, high tones become progressively more involved. The attacks of vertigo associated with Ménière's disease usually abate as hearing loss in the affected ear peaks.

451. The answer is D. *(Adams, ed 4. p 243.)* Gentamicin, kanamycin, and streptomycin usually give rise to hearing loss if they are going to affect the inner ear at all, but they do not typically cause vertigo. Alcohol and quinine, as well as salicylates, may produce a toxic labyrinthitis with vertigo as a prominent feature. Vertigo is also a common sequela of head trauma or whiplash injury.

452. The answer is C. *(Adams, ed 4. pp 240–241.)* Ménière's disease is an inner ear disorder. Both acoustic and vestibular systems are affected; consequently the patient has episodic vertigo with hearing loss and tinnitus that are more likely to be persistent or progressive. Amblyopia is a loss of vision and often refers to conditions in which perception is transiently lost in one eye or vision is permanently lost in one part of the visual field. Tobacco-alcohol amblyopia refers to a condition most often seen in habitual alcohol and tobacco users in which centrocecal scotomas evolve over months or years and greatly diminish visual acuity.

453. The answer is B. *(Lechtenberg, Synopsis, pp 127–128.)* Aspirin may produce tinnitus in persons usually unaffected by this problem. Patients on high doses of aspirin for rheumatoid arthritis are especially susceptible to this drug-induced tinnitus. Those patients with chronic tinnitus from acoustic trauma or Ménière's disease will find their symptoms worsen with aspirin.

454. The answer is C. *(Johnson, ed 3. pp 101–108.)* Café au lait spots characteristically occur in both type 1 and type 2 neurofibromatosis. Meningiomas, acoustic schwannomas, and other types of CNS tumors occur with these hereditary disorders, but the neurofibroma is the most common lesion. Type 1 neurofibromatosis develops with a defect on chromosome 17; type 2 with a defect on chromosome 22.

455. The answer is B. *(Lechtenberg, Synopsis, p 141.)* Schwannomas most often occur on cranial nerve VIII, but they may also develop on V, VII, IX, or X. With type 2 neurofibromatosis, bilateral tumors are more the rule than the exception. The tumors that develop on the eighth cranial nerve usually develop on the vestibular division of the nerve.

456. The answer is B. *(Adams, ed 4. p 183.)* The olfactory tract divides into medial and lateral striae. The medial stria sends fibers across the anterior commissure to the opposite hemisphere. The lateral stria terminates in the medial and cortical nuclei of the amygdaloid complex, as well as the prepiriform area. This primary olfactory cortex is in area 34 of Brodmann and is restricted to a small area on the end of the hippocampal gyrus and the uncus. This distribution of fibers makes olfaction unique among the senses in that it does not send fibers through the thalamus.

457. The answer is D. *(Adams, ed 4. p 185.)* Development of genitalia and secondary sexual characteristics during puberty and adolescence is usually negligible in boys affected by this syndrome. The olfactory defect is congenital but may be unsuspected until the hypogonadism becomes apparent. The defects responsible for both the anosmia and hypogonadism are developmental rather than acquired. Until the defect in secondary sexual characteristics becomes apparent, the affected person is usually perceived as normal.

458. The answer is D. *(Adams, ed 4. p 187.)* Much of taste is mediated by volatile molecules that are actually smelled. Agents that are especially pungent, such as ammonia, are inappropriate for testing smelling or taste because they stimulate common chemical sense, a modality mediated by neither taste nor smell receptors. The tip of the tongue is most sensitive to sweet and salt, the sides to sour, and the base to bitter.

459. The answer is D. *(Adams, ed 4. p 185.)* Anosmia is most likely to develop with head trauma if the trauma is sufficient to cause a skull fracture. If anosmia does occur in the setting of a skull fracture, it is likely to be permanent. With head trauma that does not cause a fracture, anosmia will persist in about 75 percent of cases.

460. The answer is C. *(Adams, ed 4. p 186.)* Ipsilateral optic atrophy and contralateral papilledema in association with an intracranial tumor is the Foster-Kennedy syndrome. A meningioma of the olfactory groove may produce this syndrome if it extends posteriorly to involve the ipsilateral optic nerve. Compression on the optic nerve by the tumor produces atrophy and interferes with transmission of the increased intracranial pressure down the optic sheath. The increased intracranial pressure is reflected in the papilledema apparent in the contralateral eye.

Spinal Cord and Root Disease

DIRECTIONS: Each question below contains five suggested responses. Select the **one best** response to each question.

461. With transection of the cervical spinal cord above the level of C5, the quadriplegic person will usually exhibit areflexia in the transiently flaccid limbs. This areflexia and flaccidity usually evolve into hyperreflexia and spasticity within

(A) 2 to 4 months
(B) 1 to 2 months
(C) 3 days to 3 weeks
(D) 1 to 3 h
(E) 5 to 25 min

462. Atrophy of the first dorsal interosseous muscle may indicate damage to spinal roots

(A) C5 and C6
(B) C6 and C7
(C) C7 and C8
(D) C8 and T1
(E) T1 and T2

463. The median nerve originates from spinal roots

(A) C5–T1
(B) C3–C4
(C) C5–T3
(D) C4–T2
(E) C1–C5

464. After biopsy resection of a lymph node in her neck, a 23-year-old woman noticed instability of her shoulder. Neurologic examination revealed winging of the scapula on the side of the surgery. During surgery she probably suffered damage to the

(A) deltoid muscles
(B) long thoracic nerve
(C) serratus anterior muscle
(D) suprascapular nerve
(E) axillary nerve

465. Fracture of a lumbar vertebral body usually occurs with spinal

(A) flexion
(B) extension
(C) torsion
(D) spondylolisthesis
(E) subluxation

466. If pain in the back of the head originates from compression of a spinal root, the root will usually be

(A) C1
(B) C2
(C) C3
(D) C4
(E) C5

467. Lissauer's tract (fasciculus gelatinosa) in the spinal cord is composed primarily of which of the following fiber types?

(A) Autonomic
(B) Pain
(C) Motor
(D) Proprioceptive
(E) Spindle efferent

468. An injury that cuts the right half of the spinal cord at the C4 root entry zone will produce impairment of ipsilateral pain perception for

(A) all levels below C4
(B) all levels above C4
(C) C4, C5, and C6
(D) only C4
(E) C1 through C7

469. With the C4 injury described in the previous question, position sense should be impaired

(A) ipsilaterally from the level of the injury caudally
(B) contralaterally from the level of the injury caudally
(C) ipsilaterally from the level of the injury cephalad
(D) contralaterally from the level of the injury cephalad
(E) exclusively at the level of the injury

470. In the Brown-Séquard syndrome of spinal cord hemisection, a spastic paresis develops in the muscles innervated by nerves derived from spinal roots

(A) bilaterally at the level of injury
(B) ipsilaterally at the level of injury
(C) contralaterally at the level of injury
(D) ipsilaterally below the level of injury
(E) contralaterally below the level of injury

471. Atlantoaxial subluxation may develop as a complication of advanced

(A) amyotrophic lateral sclerosis
(B) syringomyelia
(C) rheumatoid arthritis
(D) olivopontocerebellar degeneration
(E) neurofibromatosis

472. The cervical spinal root most commonly involved by a herniated intervertebral disk is

(A) C1
(B) C3
(C) C4
(D) C6
(E) C7

473. Compression of the C8 spinal root is easily confused with damage to which nerve?

(A) Ulnar
(B) Axillary
(C) Median
(D) Radial
(E) Long thoracic

474. Pain radiating to the ridge of the trapezius, the tip of the shoulder, the anterior part of the arm, the forearm, and the thumb may develop with a disk herniation between vertebrae

(A) C3 and C4
(B) C4 and C5
(C) C5 and C6
(D) C6 and C7
(E) C7 and T1

475. A patient's leg is lifted off the examining table without bending the knee while he is lying flat on his back, and pain is elicited in the back that radiates down the leg. This suggests

(A) torn quadriceps muscle
(B) aseptic necrosis of the head of the femur
(C) psoriatic arthritis of the spine
(D) pelvic inflammatory disease
(E) herniated lumbar disk

476. A centrally herniated cervical intervertebral disk may produce a progressive deficit similar to that in

(A) Parkinson disease
(B) Wilson disease
(C) Hallervorden-Spatz disease
(D) amyotrophic lateral sclerosis (ALS)
(E) Pick disease

477. Pancoast tumors may disturb spinal roots just as they exit from the spine. If these tumors do impinge on spinal roots, it is usually on roots

(A) C2–C3
(B) C4–C5
(C) C6–C7
(D) T1–T2
(E) T4–T5

478. All the following may develop with the superior thoracic aperture (thoracic outlet) syndrome EXCEPT

(A) deltoid weakness
(B) supraclavicular bruit
(C) asymmetric radial pulses
(D) weakness and wasting of the interosseus muscles
(E) hand pain

479. Spina bifida develops with

(A) failure of fusion of dorsal vertebral elements
(B) lysis of dorsal vertebral elements
(C) listhesis of ventral vertebral elements
(D) lysis of lateral vertebral elements
(E) failure of fusion of lateral vertebral elements

Spinal Cord and Root Disease

Answers

461. The answer is C. *(Adams, ed 4. p 45.)* Spinal shock is a transient phenomenon occurring with damage to fibers from upper motor neurons. The spasticity that usually develops within a few days of the spinal cord injury is presumed to represent exaggeration of the normal stretch reflexes in the limbs disconnected from upper motor neuron control. The evolution from spinal shock to spasticity is much more typical of spinal cord injuries than it is of cerebrocortical injuries, but even with cerebrocortical injuries there is usually an interval of hours to days during which limbs that eventually become hyperreflexic and spastic are hyporeflexic and flaccid.

462. The answer is D. *(Adams, ed 4. p 1068.)* The first dorsal interosseous muscle is innervated by the ulnar nerve. The fibers of the ulnar nerve reaching this muscle originate at C8 and T1 roots. If the ulnar nerve itself is the neural element injured, it is usually because of damage at the elbow where the ulnar nerve runs superficially in the groove over the ulnar condyle. All the interosseous muscles of the hand are supplied by the ulnar nerve. Complete transection of that nerve will produce interosseous wasting and impaired finger adduction and abduction. Although the lumbrical muscles are situated alongside the interosseous muscles of the hand, only two lumbricals—those on the ulnar metacarpals—are innervated by the ulnar nerve. The other two lumbricals are innervated by the median nerve. All four lumbricals insert on the extensor sheaths of the fingers and participate in extension of the digits.

463. The answer is A. *(Adams, ed 4. p 1067.)* The median nerve derives primarily from C6, with contributions from C5, C7, C8, and T1. These five spinal roots are also the principal contributors to the brachial plexus. The medial and lateral cords of the brachial plexus join together to form the median nerve.

464. The answer is B. *(Adams, ed 4. p 1067.)* Winging of the scapula most often occurs with weakness of the serratus anterior muscle. This is innervated by the long thoracic nerve, whose course starts high enough and runs superficial enough to allow injury to the nerve with deep dissection into the root of the neck. The long thoracic nerve is derived from C5, C6, and C7. Winging is elicited by having the patient push against a wall with the hands at shoulder level. With this maneuver the scapula with the weak serratus anterior will be pulled away from the back and the vertical margin of the scapula will stick out from the back. Injuries to the long thoracic nerve are usually unilateral and are often due to trauma or surgical manipulation.

465. The answer is A. *(Adams, ed 4. p 163.)* Extreme flexion of the lumbar spine is likely in automobile accidents with the person seated and in falls with the person upright. Fracture of a lumbar vertebral body may be seen in vehicular accidents when the victim is restrained during a high-speed impact by a seat belt without a shoulder harness. The rapid and extreme forward flexion of the lumbar spine may produce a variety of spine injuries, ranging from fractures to dislocations. Fractures suffered during falls in which the person is upright, such as may occur when someone jumps off a building, are usually compression fractures of the vertebral body. Fracture of the vertebral body will usually produce pain coincidental with the injury. Patients with fractures of the vertebral body that occur without trauma or with inconsequential trauma must be investigated for malignant processes, such as metastatic carcinoma, multiple myeloma, and unsuspected osteomyelitis.

466. The answer is B. *(Adams, ed 4. p 104.)* C1 has no sensory component. Most of the face and head receives its sensory supply from the trigeminal nerve. C2 carries sensory information from the skin over the back of the head and the neck. C3 compression usually produces discomfort over the shoulder region between the neck and the deltoid area.

467. The answer is B. *(Adams, ed 4. p 104.)* Lissauer's tract is in the lateral part of the dorsal root entry zone. Within it are some of the finest myelinated and unmyelinated sensory fibers. These fibers are primarily, but not exclusively, for pain perception. Pain perception is conducted to the spinal cord along myelinated A-delta and unmyelinated C nerve fibers. Lissauer's tract carries sensory fibers cephalad one to three cord levels before the sensory fibers decussate to the contralateral spinothalamic tracts.

468. The answer is C. *(Adams, ed 4. p 129.)* Some pain fibers travel a few cord segments cephalad in Lissauer's tract before crossing to the other side of the spinal cord. Hemisection of the cord will therefore produce a contralateral pain and temperature sensory loss extending caudally from a few levels below the site of injury. All the fibers that have crossed from the uninjured side of the spinal cord will be cut. Only those fibers that have not yet crossed from the side of injury will be cut.

469. The answer is A. *(Adams, ed 4. pp 129–130.)* Position sense remains uncrossed in the spinal cord. All the fibers ascending in the cord will be cut at the level of the injury. Unlike the arrangement for pain and temperature fibers, there is no decussation below the level of the medulla oblongata. Not until the brainstem do position and vibration sense fibers decussate.

470. The answer is D. *(Adams, ed 4. pp 129–130.)* The corticospinal tracts are cut with hemisection of the spinal cord. These fibers synapse with anterior horn cells ipsilateral to the side of the tract. Damage to the anterior horn cells by the hemisection injury will produce weakness and atrophy but should not produce spasticity in the muscles innervated by spinal roots originating at the level of the injury. Additional features of the Brown-Séquard syndrome include contralateral loss of pain and temperature sensation extending caudally from a few cord levels below the cord injury. Position and vibration sense will be lost on the same side of the body as the cord injury, and this deficit will extend from the level of the hemisection caudally.

471. The answer is C. *(Adams, ed 4. p 171.)* In atlantoaxial subluxation, the atlas usually slips anterior to its customary alignment with the axis. This misalignment develops with a synovitis at the atlantoaxial joint. With the atlas abnormally forward on the axis, the space available at C1 for the spinal cord is reduced, and the spinal cord may be compressed.

472. The answer is E. *(Adams, ed 4. p 172.)* There are seven cervical vertebrae, but eight cervical spinal roots. Fully 70 percent of cervical root compressions occur at C7. Another 20 percent occur at C6, and virtually all the remaining problems occur at roots C5 and C8. Disk herniation usually develops after trauma, but the trauma may appear to be relatively minor.

473. The answer is A. *(Adams, ed 4. p 172.)* The ulnar nerve is derived primarily from the C8 spinal root. The weakness developing with a C8 root or an ulnar nerve injury will include the interosseus muscles of the hand and the ulnar two lumbrical muscles. The sensory loss will be along the medial cutaneous nerve of the forearm and extend into the ulnar two digits of the hand. With the ulnar nerve lesion, there may be a characteristic splitting of sensory loss down the middle of the fourth digit. The radial aspect of the fourth digit gets sensory fibers from the median nerve.

474. The answer is C. *(Adams, ed 4. p 172.)* The spinal root compressed with pain radiating to the thumb is usually C6. This root exits between vertebrae C5 and C6 and may be impinged upon by a laterally herniated disk. Compression of root C8, which exits the spinal column between vertebrae C7 and T1, could produce pain in the ulnar two digits of the hand.

475. The answer is E. *(Lechtenberg, Synopsis, pp 105–106.)* The straight-leg-raising test helps to identify a radiculopathy in the lumbosacral region. Manipulation of the leg as described stretches the lumbar spinal roots. As the nerves are stretched, pain radiates down the leg along the dermatome supplied by the spinal root that is trapped or crushed. The lesion compressing the root need not be a herniated disk. Masses such as meningiomas, metastatic tumors, and neurofibromas may produce the same pattern of pain as a herniated nucleus pulposus.

476. The answer is D. *(Adams, ed 4. p 172.)* Parkinson, Wilson, Pick, and Hallervorden-Spatz diseases are all degenerative diseases of the brain rather than the spinal cord. ALS causes substantial, if not exclusive, damage to the spinal cord. With a centrally herniated cervical disk, the cord is progressively compressed and motor deficits may overshadow all other signs and symptoms. The pattern of weakness may be a spastic quadriplegia with the legs involved before the arms. Despite pressure on sensory pathways, the cord compression may proceed for years without focal neck pain.

477. The answer is D. *(Adams, ed 4. p 175.)* The Pancoast tumor is usually a squamous cell carcinoma arising from the superior sulcus of the lung and extending superiorly. It routinely produces a Horner syndrome of miosis, ptosis, and anhidrosis ipsilateral to the tumor, but it may also disturb the lower cervical (C8) and upper thoracic (T1–T2) root functions even before it is radiographically obvious. Root involvement usually produces numbness on the inner aspect of the arm, weakness of the intrinsic hand muscles, and pain beneath the upper scapula.

478. The answer is A. *(Adams, ed 4. p 174.)* There is no consensus on what causes the thoracic outlet syndrome, but explanations include cervical ribs, anomalous anterior scalene muscle insertions, and anomalous fascial bands at the thoracic outlet. The fundamental disturbances in this syndrome include compression of elements of the brachial plexus, the subclavian artery, and the subclavian vein. The neurologic deficits that appear include wasting and weakness of the hypothenar, interosseus, adductor pollicis, and ulnar two lumbrical muscles of the hand. Pain and paresthesias are usually chronically present over the ulnar aspects of the forearm and hand.

479. The answer is A. *(Lechtenberg, Synopsis, p 148.)* If the fusion defect in spina bifida is asymptomatic, the disorder is usually designated spina bifida occulta. Spina bifida of any sort is most common in the lumbrosacral region. It occurs much more commonly independently of the Chiari malformations than in association with them. With Chiari malformations of hindbrain formation, the affected person is at increased risk of a meningocele or myelomeningocele in association with the spina bifida.

Peripheral Neuropathy

DIRECTIONS: Each question below contains five suggested responses. Select the **one best** response to each question.

480. Excessive doses of what vitamin may produce a peripheral neuropathy?

(A) Thiamine
(B) Vitamin A
(C) Nicotinamide
(D) Pyridoxine
(E) Vitamin B_{12}

481. The patellar tendon reflex involves sensory fibers of the femoral nerve originating in spinal segments

(A) S3–S4
(B) S2–S3
(C) S1–S2
(D) L4–L5
(E) L2–L3

482. The most common cause of footdrop is compression of which of the following nerves?

(A) Sciatic
(B) Common peroneal
(C) Posterior tibial
(D) Sural
(E) Obturator

483. All the following may cause a footdrop and steppage gait EXCEPT

(A) Charcot-Marie-Tooth disease (peroneal muscular atrophy)
(B) poliomyelitis
(C) progressive spinal muscular atrophy
(D) L5 spinal root compression
(E) hepatolenticular degeneration

484. Of the following agents, the one most likely to produce a painful sensory peripheral neuropathy is

(A) lead
(B) manganese
(C) thallium
(D) cyanide
(E) mercury

485. Mononeuritis multiplex may routinely develop with any of the following EXCEPT

(A) diabetes mellitus
(B) temporal arteritis
(C) sarcoidosis
(D) systemic lupus erythematosus
(E) periarteritis nodosa

Peripheral Neuropathy
Answers

480. The answer is D. *(Rowland, ed 8. p 884.)* Pyridoxine overdose sufficient to produce a peripheral neuropathy is usually seen in persons taking many times the recommended daily allowance of pyridoxine in vitamin preparations. It does not develop from eating foods with high levels of pyridoxine. Excessive pyridoxine consumption is usually linked to hypochondriasis or compulsive behavior. Vitamin A excess may produce pseudotumor cerebri in children, but it does not produce a peripheral neuropathy. This hypervitaminosis is also typically the result of excessive intake of concentrated vitamin preparations rather than of foods rich in vitamin A. Deficiencies of thiamine, pyridoxine, nicotinamide, or vitamin B_{12} also may produce peripheral neuropathy. Vitamin deficiencies are a common health problem, whereas hypervitaminoses are medical oddities.

481. The answer is E. *(Adams, ed 4. p 39.)* Myotatic, or tendon stretch, reflexes require intact sensory supplies from the tendons and motor supplies to the muscles involved. The patellar tendon reflex entails contraction of the quadriceps femoris muscle group, a muscle group with four members, the vastus lateralis, vastus medialis, vastus intermedius, and rectus femoris. This reflex requires perception of stretch in the tendon stretch receptors innervated by L2 and L3. With tapping of the tendon extending from the patella to the head of the tibia, spinal reflex pathways activate contraction of the quadriceps femoris group and evoke extension of the lower leg with straightening of the knee. Damage to the motor supply to the reactive muscles must be profound before the tendon reflex will be lost completely. Corticospinal tract damage will produce hyperreflexia apparently by disinhibiting spinal cord mechanisms.

482. The answer is B. *(Adams, ed 4. p 97.)* Dorsiflexion of the foot is controlled primarily by the anterior tibial muscle. The deep peroneal nerve supplies this muscle and arises from the common peroneal nerve just below the knee. Compression of the common peroneal nerve is especially likely where it crosses the head of the fibula. A sciatic nerve injury may also produce footdrop, but this is much less common than peroneal nerve injury. During a lumbar laminectomy, spinal roots to the sciatic nerve are occasionally stretched and a transient or persistent footdrop ensues. The common peroneal nerve is more vulnerable than the sciatic because of its superficial location as it wraps around the head of the fibula just below the lateral aspect of the knee. Trauma to the side of the lower leg just below the knee may crush the nerve. The deep peroneal nerve has predominantly motor elements. Damage to the nerve may produce some loss of sensation on the dorsum of the foot between the first and second toes, but many injured persons do not even realize they have lost sensation over this small patch of skin.

483. The answer is E. *(Adams, ed 4. p 97.)* Motor neuron disease or peripheral neuropathy may evoke a steppage gait in which the patient is obliged to lift the foot abnormally far from the ground. What appears to be exaggerated flexion of the hip and knee is adopted to prevent the toes from catching on the ground. This gait disturbance compensates for failure of dorsiflexion of the feet when the patient has loss of strength in the anterior tibial muscles. Steppage gait also develops in persons with some types of muscular dystrophy. In persons with this disorder, direct injury to muscles, rather than nerves, produces the problems with dorsiflexion and eversion of the foot responsible for a steppage gait. Hepatolenticular degeneration (Wilson disease) produces gait changes, but they are reminiscent of Parkinson disease in most patients.

484. The answer is C. *(Adams, ed 4. p 831. Gilman, Disorders, pp 322–323.)* Thallium poisoning may produce hair loss, stupor, gastrointestinal distress, seizures, and headaches, as well as a painful, symmetric, primarily sensory neuropathy. Lead often produces a peripheral neuropathy in adults, but it is a motor neuropathy. Professional painters exposed to lead-based paints for years characteristically developed a wristdrop as a toxic effect of the lead they absorbed. Manganese is also a toxin, but long-term exposure to this metal may produce parkinsonism rather than a sensory neuropathy. Cyanide was long regarded as the cause of an optic neuropathy, but this lethal toxin has probably been unjustly ascribed this capability. Mercury poisoning may produce a sensory neuropathy, but it is generally associated with paresthesias rather than dysesthesias.

485. The answer is B. *(Adams, ed 4. pp 679–1047.)* Diabetes mellitus is the most common cause of mononeuritis multiplex. In this disorder individual nerves are transiently disabled. The neuropathy usually develops over the course of minutes to days, and the recovery of function may require weeks to months. Various rheumatoid diseases and sarcoidosis produce similar clinical pictures, but temporal arteritis does not typically lead to this type of neuropathy. A vascular lesion is believed to be the most common basis for this type of neuropathy. If the giant cell arteritis seen with temporal arteritis does cause a neuropathy, it is an optic neuropathy with resultant blindness. Unlike the peripheral nerve injuries developing with mononeuritis multiplex, this ischemic optic neuropathy of temporal arteritis produces irreversible injury to the affected cranial nerve. The patient who loses vision as part of temporal arteritis does not recover it.

Management

DIRECTIONS: Each question below contains five suggested responses. Select the **one best** response to each question.

Questions 486–487

A 32-year-old woman with alcoholism and cocaine use dating back at least 10 years came to the emergency room after 48 h of recurrent vomiting and hematemesis. She reported abdominal discomfort that preceded her vomiting by a few days. For at least 36 h she had been unable to keep ethanol in her stomach. Intravenous fluid replacement was started while she was being transported to the emergency room, and while in the emergency room she complained of progressive blurring of vision. Over the course of an hour she became increasingly disoriented, ataxic, and dysarthric.

486. The most likely explanation for her rapid deterioration is

(A) dehydration
(B) hypomagnesemia
(C) Wernicke's encephalopathy
(D) hypoglycemia
(E) cocaine overdose

487. Emergency administration of what medication is appropriate in this clinical setting?

(A) Glucose
(B) Magnesium sulfate
(C) Pyridoxine
(D) Cyanocobalamin
(E) Thiamine

488. The drug of choice for the treatment of infantile spasms is

(A) phenytoin (Dilantin)
(B) phenobarbital
(C) carbamazepine (Tegretol)
(D) divalproex sodium (Depakote)
(E) adrenocorticotropic hormone (ACTH)

489. Complications of ethosuximide (Zarontin) treatment include all the following EXCEPT

(A) paradoxical seizures with toxicity
(B) bone marrow aplasia
(C) acute allergic reactions
(D) systemic lupus erythematosus
(E) nephrotic syndrome

490. The 6-month-old child who develops a febrile seizure should be investigated with a spinal tap because

(A) all febrile seizures justify spinal taps
(B) most febrile seizures are from bacterial infections
(C) febrile seizures cause increased intracranial pressure that must be relieved by withdrawing CSF
(D) intrathecal antiepileptics must be given
(E) children this age may have meningitis with no manifestations other than fever and seizures

491. The antiepileptic most strongly linked with defects in neural tube closure is

(A) phenytoin
(B) divalproex sodium
(C) carbamazepine
(D) phenobarbital
(E) ethosuximide

492. Which of the following antiepileptics is strictly contraindicated during pregnancy because of its unacceptable teratogenicity?

(A) Trimethadione
(B) Phenytoin
(C) Carbamazepine
(D) Lorazepam
(E) Phenobarbital

493. With hyperprolactinemia, drug treatment is feasible with

(A) thyroxine (Synthroid)
(B) chlorpromazine (Thorazine)
(C) adrenocorticotropic hormone (ACTH)
(D) luteinizing hormone (LH)
(E) bromocriptine (Parlodel)

494. The hypersomnolence that may develop with myotonic muscular dystrophy is usually managed with

(A) phenytoin (Dilantin)
(B) phenobarbital
(C) fluoxetine (Prozac)
(D) methylphenidate (Ritalin)
(E) quinidine

495. Acute herniation of an intervertebral disk will require emergency surgery if

(A) the disk is laterally herniated at C7
(B) the disk is causing radicular pain
(C) the cauda equina is being crushed
(D) a thoracic disk is involved
(E) the filum terminale is displaced

496. Persons with gastrointestinal problems who develop signs of parkinsonism should be asked specifically about exposure to

(A) ranitidine (Zantac)
(B) antacids (Maalox)
(C) diazepam (Valium)
(D) metoclopramide (Reglan)
(E) calcium carbonate

497. Dopamine agonists are useful in managing patients with Parkinson disease and include such drugs as

(A) trihexyphenidyl (Artane)
(B) L-dopa/carbidopa (Sinemet)
(C) pergolide (Permax)
(D) benztropine (Cogentin)
(E) amantadine (Symmetrel)

498. Selegiline (Eldepryl), also known as deprenyl, has been introduced into the treatment of Parkinson disease on the assumption that it can

(A) replace dopamine stores
(B) slow neuronal loss in the substantia nigra
(C) enhance synapse formation in the basal ganglia
(D) reduce the adverse effects of dopaminergic drugs
(E) activate alternative pathways for dopamine synthesis

499. The most effective means to abort a cluster headache is

(A) inhaled 100% oxygen
(B) sublingual nitroglycerin
(C) oral methysergide
(D) oral propranolol
(E) dihydroergotamine suppository

500. The drug of choice for the management of complex partial seizures is

(A) phenobarbital
(B) phenytoin (Dilantin)
(C) carbamazepine (Tegretol)
(D) primidone (Mysoline)
(E) methsuximide (Celontin)

Management

Answers

486. The answer is C. *(Lechtenberg, Synopsis, pp 154–155.)* Wernicke's encephalopathy is a potentially fatal consequence of thiamine deficiency, a problem for which this woman was at risk by virtue of being an alcoholic. When she came to the emergency room, intravenous fluids were started that probably contained glucose. The stress of a large glucose load will abruptly deplete the central nervous system of the little thiamine it had available and will precipitate the sort of deterioration evident in this woman. Features characteristic of a Wernicke's encephalopathy include deteriorating level of consciousness, autonomic disturbances, ocular motor problems, and gait difficulty. The autonomic disturbances may include lethal hypotension or profound hypothermia. Hemorrhagic necrosis in periventricular gray matter will be evident in this woman's brain if she dies. The mamillary bodies are especially likely to be extensively damaged.

487. The answer is E. *(Lechtenberg, Synopsis, pp 154–155.)* Without rapid replacement of thiamine stores, the patient with acute Wernicke's encephalopathy may die. Usually 50 to 100 mg of thiamine are given intravenously immediately. This is followed over the course of a few days with supplementary thiamine injections of 50 to 100 mg. Without thiamine, the patient will develop periaqueductal and mamillary body lesions, which will be clinically apparent as autonomic failure. With chronic thiamine deficiency, neuronal loss occurs in alcoholic persons at least partly because of this relative vitamin deficiency. Purkinje and other cells in the cerebellar vermis will be lost to so dramatic an extent that gross atrophy of the superior cerebellar vermis will be evident.

488. The answer is E. *(Johnson, ed 3. pp 26–28.)* Conventional antiepileptic drugs have little or no effect on the seizures and subsequent retardation typically seen with infantile spasms. ACTH and corticosteroids may suppress seizure activity in these infants and may improve the profoundly abnormal EEG patterns that develop with infantile spasms. Even with ACTH treatment, 85 to 90 percent of children with infantile spasms develop retardation. This mode of therapy is fraught with complications. Children on ACTH for more than a few weeks become increasingly cushingoid. Excessive weight gain, skin eruptions, and hyperglycemia are common problems in infants treated with this hormone. Hypertension and disturbances of growth and development may also occur.

489. The answer is A. *(Johnson, ed 3. pp 33–36.)* Phenytoin may cause seizures at toxic levels, but this is not an expected consequence of ethosuximide toxicity. As with most antiepileptics, excessively high levels of ethosuximide may produce ataxia and sedation. The bone marrow depression, nephrotic syndrome, and lupus reactions that occur in some patients exposed to this drug are rare and quite unpredictable. Ethosuximide is usually used to manage generalized absence seizures in children. It is often used in children under 10 years of age with this seizure type because divalproex sodium, the antiepileptic considered by many to be the drug of choice for generalized absence seizures, has a disturbing rate of hepatic complications in this young group of patients. The hepatotoxicity of divalproex sodium is most evident before the age of 2 years, but in most of the children who develop lethal complications with this drug, congenital problems other than epilepsy suggest they are inappropriate candidates for divalproex sodium. Many physicians use phenobarbital to treat seizure disorders in children under 2 years of age, but psychomotor delays, irritability, and other behavioral problems induced by phenobarbital make it a poor alternative to other antiepileptics.

490. The answer is E. *(Johnson, ed 3. p 30.)* Between birth and 1 year of age, what appears to be a simple febrile seizure may actually be a seizure provoked by a bacterial meningitis. The agents most likely to be responsible are *Haemophilus influenzae* and *Enterococcus coli*. Both require rapid diagnosis and early treatment if the child is to survive. *E. coli* is unlikely after the newborn period. Both infections require CSF examination for the diagnosis. Even though the child may not have substantial neck stiffness, the fluid will typically reveal a glucose content less than two-thirds the serum level, elevated WBC count, and an increased protein content. The responsible organism may be isolated and cultured, but treatment of the meningitis should begin before the organism is characterized. A delay of hours in treatment may be lethal. Intravenous antibiotics should be started as soon as there is convincing evidence that febrile seizures are secondary to a bacterial meningitis. The drug chosen should be the one most effective against the most probable organism. The child's age, exposure, and symptomatology must all be considered in deciding what organism is most likely responsible for the infection.

491. The answer is B. *(Lechtenberg, Seizure, pp 174–175.)* The incidence of defects in neural tube closure is small with any antiepileptic, but it is most unequivocally increased with divalproex sodium (Depakote). The mother must take the medication during the first trimester of pregnancy to increase the risk of this birth defect in the child. Fetal exposure probably must occur during the first month of embryonic development. That is the time when the embryonic neural tube forms and closes off from the amniotic fluid. The neural tube defects seen include meningoceles and myelomeningoceles in the lumbosacral region. In the former, spinal tissue does not extend into the outpouching onto the back, and in the latter it does. With both types of defect in neural tube closure the patient has an associated spina bifida. Patients with meningoceles of the lumbosacral spine are at high risk of being paraplegic. Those with myelo-meningoceles invariably have problems with leg strength and bladder and bowel control.

492. The answer is A. *(Lechtenberg, Seizure, pp 184–185.)* Trimethadione was popular for the control of generalized absence seizures. The types of birth defects it causes are similar to those seen with other antiepileptics, but the frequency of defects in exposed children is much higher than that in children exposed to the four other antiepileptics listed. Those congenital defects include cleft palate, cleft face, ventricular septal defects, polydactyly, and hip dislocations. Trimethadione is not considered an acceptable alternative to the other antiepileptics listed and is no longer available in the United States. Birth defects with exposure to any antiepileptic are more likely if the mother takes a combination of antiepileptics during the pregnancy. The long-lived practice of combining phenytoin and phenobarbital to manage seizures produced many of the impaired children who were subsequently designated as having the fetal hydantoin syndrome. This name arose from the class of drugs to which phenytoin belongs. The cleft palate, cleft face, ventricular septal defect, and polydactyly described as part of the fetal hydantoin syndrome are more legitimately designated as components of the fetal antiepileptic syndrome. Despite their hazards to the fetus, the dangers of seizures to both the fetus and the mother during pregnancy require the continued use of these drugs throughout pregnancy. The drug chosen must be one that controls seizures and exposes the fetus to the least risk of teratogenicity. For many women, carbamazepine is a reasonable antiepileptic for use during pregnancy.

493. The answer is E. *(Lechtenberg, Synopsis, pp 141–142.)* Bromocriptine is useful with prolactin-secreting pituitary adenomas because this dopamine agonist depresses serum prolactin levels and inhibits tumor growth in many cases. Bromocriptine is a derivative of the ergot alkaloids. It probably acts directly on tumor cells to inhibit their growth and activity.

494. The answer is D. *(Johnson, ed 3. pp 400–402.)* Myotonic dystrophy causes abnormal muscle function and weakness, as well as more systemic traits, such as testicular atrophy and baldness. Dextroamphetamine, as well as methylphenidate, is helpful with the hypersomnolence associated with this disorder, but it is generally considered to have a higher abuse potential than methylphenidate. Methylphenidate has been used extensively to manage hyperactivity in children with minimal brain dysfunction. Tricyclic compounds, including imipramine and amitriptyline, also have been used for the hypersomnolence of myotonic dystrophy with some success, but the basis for their effectiveness is not understood. These antidepressants may act primarily by reducing the social withdrawal that accompanies other personality changes that are evident as myotonic dystrophy progresses. The cause of the excessive sleeping seen with myotonic dystrophy is unknown.

495. The answer is C. *(Adams, ed 4. p 176.)* Surgery may eventually be necessary with any intervertebral disk herniation, but with acute, massive cauda equina injury, surgery must be performed before the deficits are irreversible. Signs of cauda equina compression will include loss of bladder and bowel control and paraparesis or paraplegia. An acutely evolving focal motor deficit in the legs, such as a footdrop, associated with sphincter dysfunctions is justification for emergency laminectomy and disk resection. Preoperative studies should be obtained to be sure that the responsible lesion is disk herniation. Metastatic cancers, such as prostate and breast carcinoma, may imitate acute disk herniations. Establishing the identity of the lesion is important because many tumors are better managed with high-dose corticosteroids and radiation therapy than with surgery. Osteomyelitis of the vertebral body may also produce cauda equina compression, but a decompressive laminectomy is usually indicated with focal infections of this sort to maximize the recovery achieved with antibiotic therapy.

496. The answer is D. *(Adams, ed 4. p 901.)* Metoclopramide is used increasingly after gastrointestinal surgery to manage nausea and other signs of gastrointestinal irritability. Although most physicians do ask about exposure to reserpine-like medications or phenothiazines, other drugs that may cause parkinsonism in susceptible persons are sometimes overlooked. Antacids and benzodiazepines would not be expected to produce signs of parkinsonism.

497. The answer is C. *(Lechtenberg, Synopsis, p 78.)* A dopamine agonist is a drug that acts on the dopamine receptor. L-Dopa is not a dopamine agonist but a dopamine precursor. L-Dopa is converted to dopamine after it enters the CNS. Benztropine is an anticholinergic drug, and amantadine is an antiviral agent that reduces parkinsonism in some patients. The mechanism by which amantadine has its effect is unknown. There are currently three types of dopamine receptors identified in the brain: D1, D2, and D3. D3 seems to be primarily responsible for the psychiatric effects of dopaminergic drugs. An ideal dopamine agonist for the management of Parkinson disease would be one that acts primarily at the D2 receptor and has no effect at all at the D3 receptor. Besides pergolide, other dopamine agonists currently available include bromocriptine (Parlodel) and lisuride (Dopergin).

498. The answer is B. *(Johnson, ed 3. pp 250–251.)* Selegiline (deprenyl) was used in patients with Parkinson disease because it was believed to act as an antioxidant. By interfering with free-radical formation and activity in the substantia nigra cells, this drug was deemed useful as a modulator of intracellular reactions that seemed to be destroying dopamine-producing neurons. That it truly acts in this way or by a closely related mechanism is still unestablished. It appears to have monoamine oxidase–inhibiting activity and it is metabolized to an amphetamine-like by-product. Patients taking selegiline do have a slower short-term deterioration than patients with Parkinson disease who are left untreated, but the reason for this slower deterioration is unknown. Alpha-tocopherol (vitamin E) has been used with selegiline in some trials because it too is believed to eliminate free radicals and destructive oxidants that arise in substantia nigra neurons.

499. The answer is A. *(Johnson, ed 3. p 75.)* Oxygen may terminate the headache within minutes. Some physicians recommend inhaling 4 L/min of 100% oxygen by mask as soon as signs of an impending headache develop. This has prompted many sufferers of cluster headache to keep a cylinder of compressed oxygen at home during the season when they are most prone to develop such headaches. Cluster headaches usually occur at night when the patient is asleep, and so access to effective treatment during the headache is usually practical— the patient does not need to transport an oxygen tank during the day. Methysergide is effective in preventing cluster headache for many persons, but it does rarely cause the worrisome adverse effect of fibrosis. Although retroperitoneal, pulmonary, and endocardial fibroses are always mentioned in discussions of methysergide's adverse effects, they are rarely observed. Sublingual nitroglycerin may in fact trigger a headache and is not recommended for patients with migraine or cluster headaches. Propranolol is a beta-adrenergic blocking agent that is useful in the prophylaxis of some vascular headaches, but it is generally deemed of no value in aborting a cluster headache. Dihydroergotamine suppositories may abort some vascular headaches, but they do not have as obvious an effect in cluster as in classic or common migraine syndromes.

500. The answer is C. *(Lechtenberg, Seizure, pp 174–176.)* Divalproex sodium (Depakote) has appeared to be as effective and as well tolerated as carbamazepine in some persons with complex partial seizures, but divalproex sodium is usually considered the drug of choice for generalized seizures. Phenytoin is nearly, if not just as, effective as carbamazepine and divalproex sodium for complex partial seizures, but its adverse effects, such as gingival hyperplasia and sedation, make it less attractive to many patients. This is especially true for young women who are concerned about the small but real risk of increased birth defects fostered by phenytoin. Coarsening of facial features and darkening of facial and limb hair are also unacceptable side effects of phenytoin for many patients. Divalproex sodium also may cause cosmetic problems, such as hair loss and weight gain, and has greater teratogenicity than carbamazepine. For all these drugs the risks of drug-related fetal abnormalities are actually small.

Bibliography

Adams RD, Victor M: *Principles of Neurology,* 4th ed. New York, McGraw-Hill, 1989.

Davis RL, Robertson DM: *Textbook of Neuropathology.* Baltimore, Williams & Wilkins, 1985.

Gilman S, Bloedel JR, Lechtenberg R: *Disorders of the Cerebellum.* Philadelphia, FA Davis, 1981.

Gilman S, Winans SS: *Manter and Gatz's Essentials of Clinical Neuroanatomy and Neurophysiology,* 6th ed. Philadelphia, FA Davis, 1982.

Johnson RT: *Current Therapy in Neurologic Disease,* 3d ed. Philadelphia, BC Decker, 1990.

Lechtenberg R: *Multiple Sclerosis Fact Book.* Philadelphia, FA Davis, 1988.

Lechtenberg R: *Seizure Recognition and Treatment.* New York, Churchill-Livingstone, 1990.

Lechtenberg R: *Synopsis of Neurology.* Philadelphia, Lea & Febiger, 1991.

Lechtenberg R, Sher JH: *AIDS in the Nervous System.* New York, Churchill-Livingstone, 1988.

Rowland LP: *Merritt's Textbook of Neurology,* 8th ed. Philadelphia, Lea & Febiger, 1989.

Toole JF: *Cerebrovascular Disorders,* 4th ed. New York, Raven Press, 1990.

Wilson JD, Braunwald E, Isselbacher KJ, et al: *Harrison's Principles of Internal Medicine,* 12th ed. New York, McGraw-Hill, 1991.